"I've watched Jørgen in action for almost 10 years now. Besides being a super-nice guy, he's an awesome trainer! I've watched him over the years getting some of the biggest male stars ready to do their thing on film, and I have a real appreciation of his knowledge regarding the human body. Don't get me wrong—he's starting off with some good material, but the way he amps it up and fine-tunes a body is a thing of beauty. When Jørgen's clients are on his program, they look HOT! And the biggest testament to that is that they all keep coming back for more."

—SUPERMODEL CINDY CRAWFORD

"I worked out with Jørgy to prepare for both *Armageddon* and *Pearl Harbor*, and he got me in great shape."

—ACTOR BEN AFFLECK

"I tell all my actors, working out is just as important as rehearsing. It's essential that they agree to look their best on camera and follow a program that gets them ready for their close-ups. When I'm working with a new actor for a project, my first call is to Jørgen de Mey. I've counted on him numerous times to get an actor physically prepared for a role. He worked with Ben Affleck for *Armageddon* and *Pearl Harbor*, all of the actresses in *Coyote Ugly*, Tom Sizemore and Josh Hartnett for *Black Hawk Down* and *Pearl Harbor*, Keira Knightley for *King Arthur*, and Jerry O'Connell for *Kangaroo Jack*. Whether it's rapid weight loss for George Dzundza in *Crimson Tide* or changing Ben Affleck's body shape from *Chasing Amy* to *Armageddon*, Jørgen's the one I count on to make it all happen."

—PRODUCER JERRY BRUCKHEIMER

"I was told to work out with Jørgen by my employer, movie producer Jerry Bruckheimer. I didn't feel I needed personal training at the time, but I was wrong. What I learned from Jørgen will keep me in shape for the rest of my life. All that being said, any time I'm on the beach and a girl mentions how in shape I am, I know I have Jørgen to thank. That sounds weird, but it's true."

—ACTOR JERRY O'CONNELL

"As a comedy writer, I spend too much time sitting around and eating crap, and by the end of the TV season, I'm usually in horrible shape. Not only was Jørgen able to get me back into condition in a month, but with his program I was able to get through production this year without the same roller-coaster ride. It's not just working out, it's a mindset that helps you maintain a condition you're happy with."

—CREATOR/PRODUCER BILL LAWRENCE
SPIN CITY AND *SCRUBS*

"Jørgen has changed my life. I have never looked or felt better. My goal was to get stronger and leaner, and I have surpassed my expectations, both physically and mentally. I am living a healthy lifestyle by incorporating Jørgen's philosophies on training and diet. It works! And now I can't live without my Jørgen!"

—ACTRESS BRIDGET MOYNAHAN

"I have known Jørgen for about 15 years, and have watched a young man with great ambition achieve success through hard work, honesty, and loyalty. He is an inspiration to his clients—some of the most important people in the motion picture industry, including Jerry Bruckheimer and Robert Towne. I wouldn't hesitate for one moment to recommend him to any of my clients."

—AGENT FRED SPECKTOR
CREATIVE ARTIST AGENCY

"After many years of training on my own, working out with Jørgen helped me break through the burnouts and plateaus that have haunted me in the past. With him, I found myself going to the next level of conditioning and fitness. Jørgen teaches that there's nothing easy or quick to realizing one's potential. He doesn't believe in fads or false promises, but rather in counseling his clients to set long-term goals and then inspiring them to achieve them."

—DIRECTOR/PRODUCER GARY FLEDER
RUNAWAY JURY AND *DON'T SAY A WORD*

THE
ACTION
HERO
BODY

THE
ACTION
HERO
BODY

THE
COMPLETE WORKOUT SECRETS
FROM
HOLLYWOOD'S TOP TRAINER

JØRGEN DE MEY
WITH SCOTT HAYS

RODALE

Notice

The information in this book is meant to supplement, not replace, proper exercise training. All forms of exercise pose some inherent risks. The editors and publisher advise readers to take full responsibility for their safety and know their limits. Before practicing the exercises in this book, be sure that your equipment is well-maintained, and do not take risks beyond your level of experience, aptitude, training, and fitness. The exercise and dietary programs in this book are not intended to substitute for any exercise routine or dietary regimen that may have been prescribed by your doctor. As with all exercise and dietary programs, you should get your doctor's approval before beginning.

Mention of specific companies, organizations, or authorities in this book does not imply endorsement by the author or publisher, nor does mention of specific companies, organizations, or authorities imply that they endorse this book, its author, or the publisher. Internet addresses and telephone numbers given in this book were accurate at the time it went to press.

Photographs by Per Bernal

Book design and illustrations by Christopher Rhoads

Library of Congress Cataloging-in-Publication Data
Mey, Jørgen de.
    The action hero body : the complete workout secrets from hollywood's top trainer / Jørgen de Mey with Scott Hays.
        p.   cm.
    Includes bibliographical references and index.
    ISBN-13 978–1–57954–910–7 hardcover
    ISBN-10 1–57954–910–1 hardcover
    1. Bodybuilding—Training.   2. Physical fitness.   I. Hays, Scott Robert, date.
II. Title.
GV546.M49   2005
613.7'13—dc22   2005004352

Distributed to the trade by Holtzbrinck Publishers

2   4   6   8   10   9   7   5   3   1   hardcover

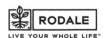

"Success is the sum of small efforts—
repeated day in and day out."

—ROBERT COLLIER,
one of America's original self-help authors

CONTENTS

PART 3:
THE ACTION HERO WORKOUT

PART 4:
THE ACTION HERO LIFE PLAN

ACKNOWLEDGMENTS

When I first visited the United States during a summer vacation from Holland some 16 years ago, I was impressed by the wide sidewalks and tall buildings, and the way that everything was open 24 hours a day. These things, which Americans take for granted, had a profound effect on me. Looking around, I felt a tremendous sense of possibility and freedom. I told myself: "I could live here, do whatever I want, create my own 'Jørgy' universe." And in many ways, since I moved to the United States, I have done just that. I now understand that this country honors people with integrity and talent, those who work hard and make the most of their prospects. That is why I want to begin these acknowledgments by giving special thanks to America, a great land of opportunity.

Writing a book about my beliefs on training, nutrition, and recuperation has long been a personal goal, and I want to thank all those who helped me to achieve it. I am particularly grateful to Scott Hays, who as-

sisted me in the writing process and who patiently listened to my re-
lentlessly enthusiastic speeches about training. I also want to thank my
agent, Scott Waxman, who "discovered" me and brought me to Rodale.
Most of all, I want to thank Zach Schisgal and Jeremy Katz at Rodale
for giving me the chance to make my dream of a book a reality.

I am grateful to Andy Pastore, chef of The White Lotus and The
Sunset Room in Los Angeles, who helped me design some tasty dishes
that are low in calories yet high in nutritional value. My appreciation
also goes to physical therapist Steve Thomas for validating my thoughts
on proper form in my exercise regimens.

In a very real sense, this book would not have been possible without
Jerry Bruckheimer, whom I met in 1990 at a time when I was just beginning to explore my capabilities as a trainer and starting to form the
philosophy behind my Action Hero training system. I could hardly
speak English back then, but evidently I got my message across, because
Jerry hired me. Today, 15 years later, he is still my most committed
client. Equally important, Jerry has introduced me to several individuals
who have become long-standing clients, and he has given me the opportunity to train numerous actors for physically demanding roles, including Josh Hartnett, Jerry O'Connell, Billy Crudup, Adam Garcia,
Bridget Moynahan, and Angelina Jolie.

Ben Affleck is the inspiration behind the title of this book. When he
signed up with me to get in shape for the movies *Armageddon* and *Pearl
Harbor,* he consistently gave 110 percent. Ben not only looked like the
hero I trained him to be in the movies but also acted like one off camera,
exhibiting the kind of strong moral and ethical behavior that all human
beings should strive to maintain in life.

Through my work, I have met some truly wonderful people, and I
am grateful to all my clients for their ongoing support and dedication.
But I especially want to acknowledge Robert and Luisa Towne, who
helped me to get established in Los Angeles. Through the years, they
have been exceptionally generous and supportive, and I feel fortunate to
count them as friends. They mean more to me than words can express.

My family in the Netherlands has always had faith in me, even when I wanted to "do my own thing" and move far from home. In particular, I am grateful to my brother, who has always been my role model—first as a brother and friend, later as a bodybuilder, and more recently, as a loving husband and father. He was my first "client," and what I learned in training him continues to inform my approach today.

I especially want to thank my wife, Angel, whom I met—and it couldn't be more perfect—in a gym. Throughout the process of writing this book, as in all of our life together, she has believed in me, helped me with my decision making, and supported my choices. She is definitely my better half. I also want to acknowledge my children: Vincent, who has taught me all the raw essentials of life, and Emma, who gives me the kisses, smiles, and hugs that just make me melt. They inspire me to do my best every day. Finally, I owe thanks to God for giving me the brain and the body that have gotten me to this point. It's been a great life so far, and I wouldn't change a thing.

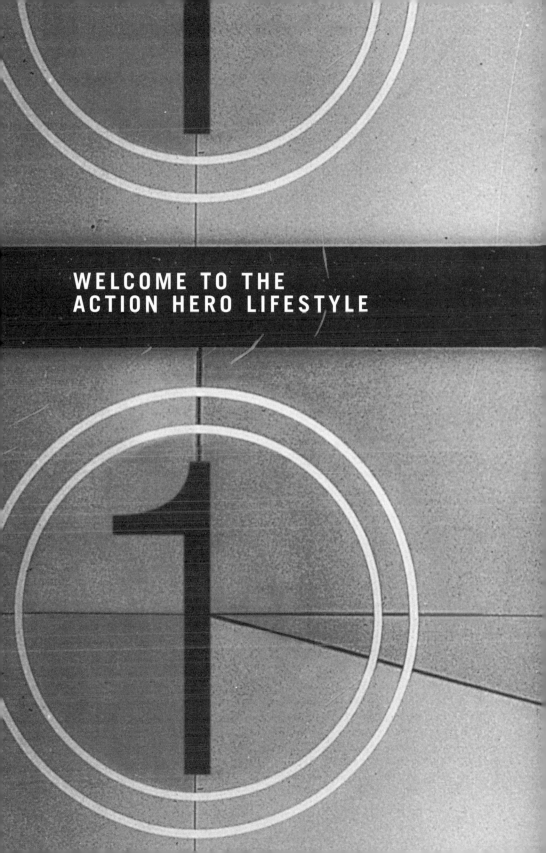
WELCOME TO THE
ACTION HERO LIFESTYLE

1

IT'S A WONDERFUL LIFE

THERE'S AN ACTION HERO in all of us. Chances are you won't believe that about yourself, but it's true. After reading this book and following the guidelines I offer in it, you'll see the proof in your own transformed physique and sense of well-being.

For more than 2 decades, I've taught and lived my "action-reaction" method of nutrition and physical training, and I've mastered it well enough to help any healthy person reach his or her personal best. It's this "best" in us that ultimately turns us into Action Heroes. I've seen it work for dozens upon dozens of people, and I've been through the process myself. I'm the living proof that it works and that it can work for you.

My own transformation began in the Netherlands, where I grew up. As a child I was always sick. My immune system couldn't guard me even from sudden changes in temperature. On a normal spring day, for instance, I'd run outside the house without a jacket and invariably catch a cold. Whenever I imposed an additional strain on my immune system, such as inadequate sleep, overexertion, or improper diet, I became an easy target for invading viruses and bacteria.

This happened too many times to count during my childhood. Finally, when I was about 12 years old, I said to myself, "This must stop! I don't want to be sick anymore!"

I decided that I had to eat better, following the guidelines my grandma taught me. "Breakfast is the most important meal of the day," she'd remind me. "Eat a sandwich with meat for lunch, and vegetables, meat, and potatoes for dinner." This was when I first realized how important a sensible diet was to becoming healthy and strong, both physically and mentally.

Without knowing where it might lead, by resolving to become healthy, I'd created a big challenge for myself. That didn't stop me, though. I was determined to succeed. The day-to-day stress and strain on my system continued—I was biking 16 miles to school every day, doing homework, doing chores around a local farm, and playing, of course. Even though I remained skinny, I became much stronger than I looked. And I was sick far less often.

I'd begun the process of becoming an Action Hero.

About this time my brother Berry became involved in boxing and then bodybuilding. He was genetically blessed in that he could build muscles quite easily with weight lifting and following a nutritionally sound diet. When I was 15, I shifted from building my body, as I'd already been doing for several years, to a more formal weight-training program like Berry's. I also got serious about understanding the role nutrition plays in increasing strength and improving health.

FOLLOW THE GUIDELINES

Media often greatly influence our attitudes about diet. Unfortunately, they often present incorrect information.

How many times have you heard that pasta, potatoes, and bread aren't good for you? The fact is, they can be great sources of energy and micronutrients when they're incorporated into a well-balanced diet. You've probably also heard that pork (the "other white meat") is healthy. People often place it in the same category as lean chicken or fish. But pork is way too high in fat and relatively low in protein. A chicken breast with no skin has just as much protein as a comparable piece of pork, but only half the calories.

Many people say they can eat whatever they want, including junk food, without ever getting fat. These individuals might burn more calories than the average person, but they're still depriving their bodies of essential building blocks in the form of usable nutrients, such as protein, complex carbohydrates, and essential fats. Their bodies will become progressively more unhealthy and less efficient as a result.

You and so many of your friends can pretty much eat whatever you want as long as the diet's tweaked to the Action Hero lifestyle.

Eat as much as you want from "good" food, but only what you need.

Let me repeat: Eat as much as you want from "good" food, but only what you *need.*

For openers, "bad" food does nothing constructive for the body. On the contrary, "bad" food is more like cancer—it slowly makes the body weaker over time, causing joint pain, fatigue, and an overall diminishment of condition and performance.

But by applying certain lifestyle adjustments—such as a healthy diet, exercise, and proper rest—you can experience better performance and a better way of life.

Or perhaps you fall into the category of people who used to be thin and able to eat anything without getting fat. But now you're in your late twenties or early thirties, and those extra 10 or 15 pounds seem to have come from nowhere and apparently plan to stick around indefinitely.

If, on the other hand, you're of the group raised on an average American diet of high calories and huge portions, you probably became fat and unhealthy at an early age. This group in particular is destined—doomed, really—to remain unhealthy for the rest of their (usually short) lives unless they take charge now and follow the guidelines outlined in this book.

With weight lifting added to my routine, my overall health improved, as did my muscle strength. Naturally my appetite increased, too, so I started eating more. However, I didn't jeopardize the beliefs my grandma had instilled in me. I just added more of the food she'd recommended: bigger breakfasts, four sandwiches at midmorning, four more in the early afternoon, a bottle of yogurt drink on the way home from school, and then a big dinner.

At this point I was changing from a boy into a man. My growth hormone and testosterone levels peaked at about the same time, and I capitalized on that by gaining 22 pounds of muscle between the ages of 17 and 18.

While coaching my brother for bodybuilding contests, I learned how to balance training with rest in conjunction with the proper foods. Berry had been my inspiration since an early age. He possessed all the Action Hero qualities: strength, passion, gentleness, healthy looks, and a great outlook on life.

When he turned 18, he trained less than a year before he took the national Mr. Iron Man junior competition, and in the same year he also took the Mr. Hercules title. At 20, he won the Grand Prix of Holland, which qualified him to compete in the Mr. Europe senior competition. He went on to win the whole show. Nobody under 21 had ever done that, other than seven-time Mr. Olympia and now California Governor Arnold Schwarzenegger.

Of course, I realized that only a handful of athletes ever manage such accomplishments. Nonetheless, we can all learn from them by studying the ways in which they reached their outstanding goals. We can learn how to harness our own strength and discipline to obtain our personal goals. This applies to all aspects of life. You don't have to be a professional to act like one. I've lived by this rule since a young age.

All through Berry's career, I continued to learn about the good and bad aspects of training and diet. I transformed from a kid who caught colds when he ran outside without a coat to a healthy man who has maintained his personal physical best for many years.

I learned that it's possible to become an Action Hero, and I'd like to help you attain this healthy goal yourself.

From Personal Best to Personal Trainer

When my brother and I came to the United States in 1989, I didn't have anything going for myself personally or professionally. I had quit my job in Holland and was starting to hate the weather and social structure there. So Berry didn't have to try very hard to convince me to come along with him.

That summer, during a cookout hosted by the Barbarian Brothers, then-young actors who starred in a late 1980s movie, *The Barbarians*, I met Jim Crabbe, vice president of William Morris Agency. Earlier, before I arrived in the United States, he'd invited me to stay at his place and even use his car until I had my feet on the ground in my new country.

He kept his word, not only about staying at his house but also about allowing me to drive his big Ford convertible. What a deal, and how nice of him to follow through on a promise like that. He was the one who made it possible for me to stay in the United States.

Not long after I arrived in Los Angeles, I landed a job as a security officer, complete with a black leather belt and handcuffs (no weapons, though). I worked the swing shift Wednesday through Sunday. It was hard work, standing on my feet, walking around for 8 hours, making civil arrests, and to be honest, I had the time of my life. The pay wasn't much, but it allowed me to get by, especially since I didn't have to pay rent. Besides, there I was, in sunny southern California. That was what mattered most.

One day my brother said to me, "Jørgy, you should be a personal trainer. You've been coaching, supporting, and motivating me for 10 years now, and I think one of your greatest strengths is that you're dedicated to helping people in the same way you'd help yourself."

Little did I know his comment would change my life forever.

Beginning that month, I went to Gold's Gym in Venice every day to study other trainers, how they worked with their clients, what they did right and, more important, what they did wrong. I got my first client shortly thereafter.

Two months later, I relocated to a tough neighborhood of Venice, not far from the gym. I decided at that point to concentrate exclusively on personal training. It was, after all, what I knew best and loved the most.

With that in mind, I met with a trainer who worked with a lot of Hollywood celebrities, and he employed me to train some of his clients. He also helped me understand the benefits of superset-oriented work-

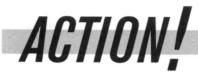

Action Hero: Jerry Bruckheimer

Career accomplishments: Film producer known for dozens of successful action and adventure movies. Along with his partner, the late Don Simpson, Jerry produced 15 Academy Award–nominated films. Their films also won two Oscars for Best Song, four Grammys, and three Golden Globes. Their top hits included *Beverly Hills Cop* and *Top Gun.* After his partner died at 51, Jerry went on to produce *Con Air, Armageddon, Pearl Harbor, Coyote Ugly, Pirates of the Caribbean,* and *National Treasure,* among others. He's also produced for television, notably the popular *CSI, Without a Trace,* and *The Amazing Race.*

Physical goals: To maintain muscularity, strength, flexibility, and cardiovascular condition.

Training program: Superset-oriented workouts in accordance with the Action Hero training system, and abdominal work with stretching.

Results: Slender, athletic build with great strength and endurance in lower and upper body.

Jerry has been my most committed trainee over the years. We share a lot of beliefs about training and diet—and what those two things together can mean to one's health, other than just being strong.

outs and circuit training. (A superset, by the way, is nothing more than two or more exercises performed one after the other. Typically, these exercises work opposing muscles: back and chest, or biceps and triceps. This allows you to work one muscle group while resting the other.) I was expanding the variety of workouts for my clients and had a suitable routine for every person I trained, helping them aim toward the goals and results they sought.

I loved the challenge of tapping into other people's potentials, goals, and needs. It seemed like I had a natural feeling for this type of work—an instinct, a gift. I was more than ever convinced that this was the right career for me.

Jerry has been training according to a 4-day schedule. Monday: back, rear delts, and biceps heavy and triceps light; Tuesday: chest, side delts, and triceps heavy and biceps light; Thursday: legs and calves; Friday: shoulders heavy and biceps/triceps light. Besides working out with me, he plays hockey and practices hockey on "off" days. With this 4-day schedule, he's maintained his overall body strength, and that's kept him stable on the ice.

When you ask him how he can work so hard, he'll give you the same reasons and explanations detailed in this book.

Even when Jerry is on the road, he finds the time to work out, following a circuit schedule—which I have explained in this book. Every 2 or 3 days, he'll train his back, chest, delts, biceps, and triceps on the same day for four or five rotations, 12 to 15 reps each set, and with weights set at around 70 percent of his peak capacity (that is, one exercise for each muscle group). This keeps his muscles conditioned and strong, and it also keeps his entire body in optimal condition.

Hard and heavy training helps maintain muscle tone and strength. Plus, the integration of cardiovascular conditioning, such as riding a stationary bike or ice skating, into a workout program helps one's lung capacity for better, deeper breathing.

During this time I met Jerry Bruckheimer, a good-looking, healthy, and trim man. I had no clue about the entertainment business, but I soon learned he wasn't a man of many words. He apparently liked the workouts and what I had to say about nutrition and bodybuilding, and he thanked me at the end of the 10 days when my employer, his own trainer, returned.

One afternoon, I came home and listened to a message on the answering machine: "Jerry Bruckheimer and Don Simpson want you to come down to Paramount Pictures to meet with them." Before that meeting, I found out more about the movie business and, specifically, those two individuals. Then I put on my best jeans, shirt, and cowboy boots, and off I went.

I was nervous as I walked into their office at Paramount Pictures, though I tried to look as composed as I could. I stopped halfway between Don's and Jerry's desks. Everything seemed to move in slow motion, and then Don said, "We, Jerry and I, want you to be our trainer."

At last, I thought, the moment of truth.

I've trained Jerry for 15 years now, and he's referred me to numerous clients, including Ben Affleck, Faye Dunaway, Josh Hartnett, Robert Towne, Bridget Moynahan, Tom Sizemore, Jerry O'Connell, Maria Bello, Piper Perabo, and Jeremy Irons. As he's done so many times before, he discovered a talent—in my case, an ability to be a personal trainer—and helped me make the most of it. He gave me a great opportunity, and I took it.

2

6 WEEKS WITH BEN AFFLECK

ON A BEAUTIFUL HAWAIIAN morning in the little village of Kailua, on the island of Oahu, I stood on a beach preparing myself physically and mentally for the first day with my new client: A-list Action Hero superstar Ben Affleck. The producer and director of the movie *Pearl Harbor* had hired me to help Ben get in optimal shape before they started filming in 6 weeks.

When Ben joined me on the beach, he was still recovering from jet lag. I decided then and there that we should take it easy the first time out, so we began jogging slowly. This was fine with me, because I would have recommended a moderate pace in any case. As with every new workout regimen, it's important to start out slowly. Even if you think the workout is insignificant, your body might react differently, especially the next day. So always start with moderate exercise, then see how you feel right after the workout, a few hours later, and the next day. If you're feeling great, go ahead and increase the intensity the next time you work out.

About 10 minutes into the jog, I decided we should speed it up a little. After about 20 minutes, we were running at a good pace, and I sensed that Ben was pleased to find himself in better condition than he'd anticipated.

The first step toward your Action Hero goal is the same no matter who you are: Stop thinking about it and actually start doing it. Ben needed to get in shape so he'd look his best on screen (which he did, by the way). And he had to do it in record time—about 6 weeks. Once a person begins adhering to a plan of diet and exercise, he'll be working toward his ultimate goal of a lean, muscular, and healthy physique.

That morning, after my first run with Ben, I checked on the breakfast table where all the foods I'd requested the night before had been set out. The producer had arranged for Ben to have his own chef, and although that made things easier for him during the film shoot, his diet would be the same one I recommend in this book—whole foods in well-balanced combinations and all easy to prepare. Every night the chef and I discussed the menu for the next day. She prepared tasty meals with fresh ingredients but stayed within the program's guidelines.

After breakfast we went over the program's specifics, including how I planned to intensify the aerobic activity and weight-lifting sessions. It was important that Ben become stronger and healthier each day because of the progressively intensifying daily routine and the program's tight deadline.

After some downtime following breakfast, we drove to a gym in the little village of Kailua. From the parking lot outside, you could tell that the gym was upstairs, because it was the only place with the windows open. All the other businesses had their windows shut tight and the air-conditioning running full blast. We walked up the wooden staircase and were surprised by the pictures on the wall. Loads of celebrities had worked out at this little gym.

"Aloha," called the muscular man behind the counter. He had a big smile on his face, probably because he knew another celebrity photo would soon be added to the collection on his wall.

The gym itself was clean and well-ventilated. I was surprised to find such fine equipment in a small town like Kailua. Apparently the gym didn't have a lot of members, which was good for us. The place stayed empty from the time that we arrived, and we could exercise without distractions or delays.

I outlined the workout plan for Ben, beginning with a 5-minute warmup on the bike. It's important to start with the bike or some other cardiovascular machine to "wake up" the body and stimulate bloodflow. This in turn ensures that your muscles and joints will receive the nutrients they need during the workout. We'd follow that with an upper body circuit training. That way we could figure out where Ben was in terms of muscle strength, stamina, and overall endurance. We'd polish up his form where needed and finish off with a short, intense abdominal routine.

An hour later, we were back downstairs in the parking lot, still sweaty and pumped. It's no big deal in Hawaii to walk out like that, because the heat and moisture won't allow your body to cool off too quickly. Rather than working out in a cold, air-conditioned environment, it's better to train in a cool to warm, well-ventilated one. Your muscles respond better when they're warm and supplied with lots of oxygen, which you won't get in a cold room sealed like a refrigerator.

The sun hovered overhead. The view, with the lagoon on one side of us and the white-sand beach and sea on the other, was breathtaking. As we drove home, I pointed out a restaurant at the end of a wooden bridge and suggested we could have steak and fresh ahi there on the special-meal weekends. These meals help break up the rigid weekly routine, and although they might have more calories than what you'd eat during the week, they're nutritious and at the same time enjoyable.

Besides, healthy alternatives are always better than, say, fast-food restaurants. Even though fast foods aren't really that tasty, you start craving them when you have a good appetite all the time. And because you're not allowed to eat them on this particular program, you want them even more. Instead, go for the restaurant that serves good, wholesome food. Even a gourmet pizza is better than the one delivered to your front doorstep.

When we got back to the compound, I went to my room, sat down at my desk, and wrote down all the newly gathered information about Ben's workout: exercises, sets, reps, resting time, pulse response, and the workout's total direct impact.

As you follow the program outlined in this book, you might find it helpful to do the same for yourself. You'll learn about your strengths as well as areas that need improvement. You'll also be able to chart the progress you make, which will help keep you motivated.

I made a note to myself to check the indirect impact from Ben's first workout, which could have included soreness, muscle fatigue, perhaps even body exhaustion. However, I thought this last unlikely, given Ben's excellent basic condition.

After noting everything down, I went to the kitchen to check with the chef and see that the meal had been prepared according to the pro-

ALL CALORIES ARE NOT CREATED EQUAL

Let's compare the equal calories—say, about 200—in a chocolate chip cookie and a small bowl of oatmeal with fat-free milk. The oatmeal with fat-free milk is high in valuable complex carbohydrates, which supply muscle energy, and unsaturated fat to keep your metabolic processes firing on all cylinders and has relatively high levels of protein, which your body uses for brain function and to repair muscle tissue and balance other internal systems. The chocolate chip cookie will do nothing for you, except make you fat.

gram. The lunch was perfect: barbecued fish with lemon and herbs, lightly sautéed local vegetables, and a scoop of seasoned brown rice.

After lunch, I suggested to Ben that it would be prudent to take an hour-long nap. Rest helps the body regain strength for the afternoon session. Because lunch was so light, Ben would still continue burning calories fairly quickly after his workout; resting wouldn't affect his digestion or lower his metabolism. Usually it's unwise to fall asleep on a full stomach, because your body's metabolism slows down when it's at rest or asleep, and food tends to be processed and stored as fat at these times. You want to digest the food and get those nutrients to your muscles, where they'll do the most good. Naps, when you have the time to indulge in them, are best taken at midday rather than after dinner.

While Ben rested, I walked outside for a little rest and relaxation myself. The yard overlooked the ocean, and I suddenly felt like fishing. It was a good time to kick back a little. Even when you're motivated and carefully following the Action Hero plan, as I have for years, you need to take time off from it periodically to redirect your thoughts toward relaxation and enjoying life. Fishing was something I didn't usually do in L.A., and I knew the interlude would refresh my mind so that I could maintain the daily commitment of workouts and dietary guidelines required by the plan. One of my principles is to teach by example and follow the Action Hero program exactly as I expect my clients to do—even when it comes to taking some time off.

I'd bought a fishing pole in town when I'd first arrived, just in case. I didn't have any bait, but I was sure one of the friendly locals would lend me some of his.

The locals were excellent fishermen. They gave me instructions on how to bait the hook, prepare for the big throw, and finally pull the line tight so you could feel the slightest movement on the hook. A half-hour went by, but I was patient.

Finally, I noticed the tip of my pole moving slightly. I thought it was just the wind at first, but all of a sudden the movement became fierce. I yanked the pole backward and reeled in the fishing line. I couldn't believe the pressure. I'd caught big pikes back in Holland, but this felt like I was trying to pull the Titanic ashore. It must be a big fish, I thought.

"Don't worry, my friend, just reel it in." One of the locals was watching and laughing. So I did. At the end of the line was a very ugly fish, flat and gray with round, popping eyes sticking out of its head. It wasn't big, but it certainly was strong. The locals explained later that it was able to stick itself tight to the sea floor.

I released the fish and returned to the house, set the pole aside, and entered the main house through the sliding doors. Ben was already taking his supplements in the kitchen and looking at the schedule I'd drawn up for him.

For that afternoon, he had a choice of some kind of aerobic activity, in order to burn more body fat. It had to be moderate activity of consistent intensity. We could hike over the mountain ridge that overlooked the ocean and town, go for a light jog on the beach, rent one of the water bikes and pedal for about 45 minutes, or return to the gym and walk on an inclined treadmill. The important thing was to make sure that the activity wasn't too intense and that Ben's heart rate stayed around 120 to 130 beats per minute, tops.

Ben decided on a jog. Along the way, I continued to ask him questions about his life as an A-list Action Hero superstar. This little conversation of ours allowed me to check whether the activity was too intense. It wasn't, because we were able to hold a normal conversation while exercising, a good indication that we'd kept the activity right in the fat-burning target range. You can use this practical gauge yourself during your aerobic workouts to determine if you're exercising at a fat-burning rate. If you can maintain a normal conversation while exercising, you're in the right range. If you're slurring your words or out of breath, you're going too fast. Remember, moderate aerobic activity burns more fat.

For dinner that night, the chef prepared whitefish—grilled, of course—a large salad, and a platter of sautéed vegetables.

I realized that this first day was one of the best starts of any program

I'd done. Everything had gone according to plan and better. It was truly a promising first step toward reaching the 6-week goals we'd set.

Three weeks later, another actor, Josh Hartnett, threw a party down the street from us. He'd just arrived on the island for some rehearsals and to meet some of the actors working on the movie. Ben and I were invited.

I was a little alarmed at the thought of going to a party. Usually not much good can come from social events when you're on the type of program Ben and I were maintaining. Fortunately, it was an early barbecue with steak, fish, and chicken. I was particularly delighted to see that Ben had eaten his dinner and taken his supplements before leaving for the party. By sticking to his diet, as I had suggested, Ben was less likely to be tempted at the party with foods not so favorable to his health.

It had been almost 3 weeks since that first jog on the beach, and already I noticed a change in Ben's behavior. His discipline and his dedication to the program were unparalleled, and more important, his body and appearance showed the first signs of a change.

I call this stage of the Action Hero program the 3-week turnaround. It always goes like that. Give your system a few weeks to get used to the program, and you realize how previous lifestyle habits contributed to an unhealthy body. You'll still be tempted to return to the old habits, but your physical well-being and improved appearance will motivate you to stick with the program. From then on, the Action Hero plan starts to become a true lifestyle—one that you won't want to change.

Sixth Week of a 6-Week Program

Ben and I began the last week of our 6-week program and were training hard. On an average day, we'd hike in the mountains for an hour in the morning before breakfast. An hour and a half after breakfast, we'd hit the gym, and Ben would do his heaviest set, 12 reps of one-arm rows using 85-pound weights and 8 reps of the dumbbell press on a flat bench, using 75-pound weights. On leg days, he'd do 15 reps of leg presses, using about 500 pounds.

Incredible! He'd started with half those weights on these particular exercises and fewer reps per set.

After the weights, if we didn't do a 15-minute cardio test on the bike (see the Stage One workout in chapter 7), set at level 12 at 90 to 100 rpms, we'd hike or jog in the late afternoon or return to the gym for an hour session on the treadmill.

ACTION!

Action Hero: Ben Affleck

Career accomplishments: Began acting in feature films in 1993, when he was cast in *Dazed and Confused.* Appeared in independent films such as *Mallrats* and *Chasing Amy.* Then he and longtime friend Matt Damon took a chance together and wrote *Good Will Hunting.* It was released in 1997, and the two became instantly famous. Since then, Ben has gone on to star in hits like *Armageddon, Shakespeare in Love,* and *Pearl Harbor.*

Physical goals: To get Ben back into shape in a record 6 weeks for the movie *Pearl Harbor.* Trim body fat, increase muscularity and muscle tone, and improve overall physical condition.

Training program: This evolved from a primarily fat-burning workout (Stage Two) to a more specific Action Hero program (Stage Three). This dude is an Action Hero! Fat-burning aerobic sessions, such as jogging on the beach, kayaking, hiking, and so on were integrated wherever possible into the program.

Results: He lost 10 pounds of body fat and replaced it with well-developed shoulders and arms.

When Ben comes to me to get ready for a movie—and this was especially true for *Pearl Harbor*—we have to get him into shape quickly. I set him up with a nutrition program tailored to his needs. Its basic components are oatmeal, egg-white omelets, chicken and lean fish, rice and vegetables, and some fruit.

Day in and day out, we worked out, but if I thought Ben needed to rest for a day, I'd slow us down and we wouldn't do a darn thing. He'd get nervous, because he felt that he had to do *something*, but he always trusted me and did what I asked of him.

Finally, my time on the island was up. I'd done my job. Ben looked phenomenal, and more important, he felt incredibly healthy and strong. During the course of 6 weeks, he'd transformed his body into a true Action Hero's physique.

Along with that I draw up a supplementation program with vitamins and amino acids, and I have him maintain a workout that includes a superset weight-lifting regimen and cardiovascular activity in between the lifting. This way, he gets prepared for the intense lifting, while the improved circulation from the cardiovascular activity allows him to work his body more efficiently.

Gradually, we increase the weight in the workouts, and he needs more rest between sets. After about 2 weeks, I take the cardio intervals out of the workout and change them to aerobic activities later in the day or on a different day entirely. No matter what we do, we always integrate some abdominal work into the hard-core workouts.

Here's a blueprint of one of Ben's workouts before *Pearl Harbor:* one-arm rows with E-Z bar French presses, 8 to 12 reps at 85 to 95 percent of his capacity; lat pulldowns, still using heavy weights but no fewer than 12 reps; and overhead triceps extensions, 15 reps using lighter weight, but still at full capacity. Because this part of the workout is so hard, we finish off with biceps, two different exercises and one set at a time.

All his workouts are like that, whether they're for his back, chest, shoulders, legs, or arms. They're always strong and intense. Just like the man himself.

Intense weight lifting helps increase muscle tone. Aerobic activity (low to moderate intensity) aids in the fat-burning process.

3

ABOUT THE
PROGRAM

B *OOM!* **BACK TO REALITY. Chances are, yours, like mine, doesn't involve a beautiful island in the middle of the Pacific, where the only objective is to get in shape. For sure you can't afford a personal trainer or a personal chef who prepares all your meals.**

In fact, it's far more likely that on any given day, you're still sitting on your couch at 9:00 P.M. after a hard day's work at the office or factory. You haven't the time or energy to seriously consider the idea of getting into shape, much less actually carry it out.

But this is where I must convince you that it's possible for normal, hardworking folks to follow the Action Hero program outlined in this book. You'll reap the same great benefits that Ben Affleck did while preparing for his film in Hawaii, or that any of my other high-profile clients have over the years.

Like Ben, though, you're going to have to trust me until you see for yourself the astonishing results. The program might strike you as un-achievable at first and nothing like anything out there, but I've helped many people achieve their goals over the years using the same techniques described here.

The secret to the program is that it really is manageable. In fact, if you decide to follow this program, you'll reach a point where you might be thinking it's not working because you're doing too *little*.

For instance, as you follow through on the cardiovascular exercises described in the Action Hero plan, people might approach you in the gym and wonder what you're doing. Whatever it is, they'll notice you're not knocking yourself out on the treadmill. You tell them you're doing "The Cart."

The Cart?

Yes, it's a great exercise for people who've been doing too much cardio activity with too much intensity. I have my clients walk on a treadmill set at an incline of 10 percent for 30 to 45 minutes at a speed of 2.5 rpm. They look like they're pushing a cart in the supermarket—hence, the name. For some people, I recommend they do this twice a day on days they don't lift weights.

Likewise with my nutrition plan. I like to stress the difference between a low-carb, high-protein diet and a more sensible one with moderate carbohydrates and a normal amount of protein. A lot of people eat way too much protein for their bodies to assimilate and not enough carbs. The truth is, your body needs the carbs in moderate amounts, especially early in the day. Depriving yourself of carbs is a good way to sabotage your efforts to lose weight and get in shape. So on the Action Hero nutrition plan, you can even eat bread again and not feel guilty about it.

(continued on page 24)

THE POWER OF "THE CART"

A lot of people ask me in the gym what fat-burning machine or activity I think is best. They're almost always surprised to learn my secret weapon: Instead of performing an exercise harder, faster, and quicker, I tell them to go easier, slower, and longer. It's all about raising the heart rate and finding yourself in the fat-burning zone.

Sure, you can get on a stationary bike, elliptical machine, stairclimber, or rowing machine, but they target a specific muscle group that must work hard by itself to raise the heart rate. Why not choose a machine that works multiple muscle groups together and will help your body raise its heart rate, without specifically burning out a specific muscle group?

What do I typically suggest? The good old-fashioned walking machine or treadmill.

At the time these machines became popular, I was involved in bodybuilding and always tried to find a way to burn more fat without jeopardizing the muscle mass that's required in a major bodybuilding competition. Running would hurt my knees and ankles, and I had to go too fast to raise my heart rate, even to a mild 130 beats per minute. The stationary bike, on the other hand, would target the individual muscle groups such as the quads, and I would complain about getting skinny legs and being depleted overall without noticing any significant effect on my body's fat reserves. Doing the stairs just landed me with the same problems.

My brother was preparing for a major bodybuilding event, and he had only 10 weeks to get into major-league shape. He weighed 260 pounds, with body fat about 20 percent. In conjunction with his diet, he needed an exercise that would help him burn fat calories more efficiently. Running didn't work; neither did stairs. So I suggested he get on a treadmill. He started at low speeds, then worked up to a faster pace. But even at a faster pace his heart rate would barely break 120 beats per minute, and his ankles started to hurt.

We then dropped the speed to 2.7 and switched to an incline to simulate walking up a hill. To make a long story short, I had him do the treadmill at a speed of 2.5, an incline of 13, and while holding on to the machine. However, few of us walk while holding on to something. So I had him push himself against the machine ever so slightly, to get the upper body just a tiny bit involved. It was like he was pushing a cart, referred to now as "pushing *The* Cart." Just imagine yourself pushing a cart full of groceries up a hill.

After 20 minutes he started to sweat, but he was still strong and didn't feel any muscle fatigue. After 30 minutes he was drenched but still strong. This was exactly what I was looking for: a relatively low-impact activity with fat-burning capacity, something that wouldn't deplete the system and put too much strain on individual muscle groups.

Now every time I design a program for someone, I incorporate The Cart. You can vary the speeds to suit your needs: for example, more of a speed walk with a lower incline, although that won't target your gluteus and calves as much. Go instead with high incline if you can keep the speed low (2.3 to 2.7 miles per hour), and make long, lungelike strides while holding the machine and pretending you're pushing a cart up a hill.

My brother, by the way, went from about 20 percent body fat to a low 4 percent. His weight dropped 15 pounds, which meant that he gained muscle while he was losing fat. Not only did he burn fat more efficiently than ever before, he also burned more calories on a daily basis. Significantly more!

Now I incorporate The Cart for all my male clients who want to gain muscle and lose fat. It really works.

Let me give you a few more applications of The Cart:

1. This is a good warmup for all the upper-body workout days. You can start with a speed somewhere between 2.5 and 3 miles per hour and an incline of 5 percent. Gradually, during the first 2 minutes, work your way up as high as possible without getting dizzy. Think of it as lunges on a treadmill. Do this for 7 to 10 minutes and then take it down gradually for a 1-minute cooldown. You're ready for a kick-ass upper-body bonanza workout.

2. On days when you do only aerobic activity, give yourself a jump start and do the first 15 minutes as I described above. Then take it down to a level that will bring your heart rate to about 120 to 130 beats per minute for the remainder of the aerobic session—let's say another 20 to 30 minutes. (Even another 15 minutes will do, as a rule; your body will start burning fat only after about 20 minutes of aerobic activity.)

3. Use it as a full-fledged cardio workout. Do your regular warmup and start out with a speed of 3 miles per hour, then work your way up to an incline of 13 to 15 percent. Find your 85 percent target heart rate and cruise at that rate for 20 to 40 minutes. After you're done with the high-intensity "pushing The Cart," take the treadmill *gradually* down to zero incline. Make sure you take about 2 to 3 minutes to cool down.

Vitamin and mineral supplementation and amino acids are very important to the plan as well. They allow your body to recover more quickly. I've dedicated an entire chapter to this concept (see chapter 6).

The program itself is based around a 24-hour cycle. During each cycle, you exercise and eat in specified amounts in order to keep your metabolism functioning at its optimal rate. You follow the program to the letter for 5 days a week, usually Monday through Friday, and on the weekends you get to treat yourself to a steak or some other favorite food.

What's not to like?

The 3-week turnaround that Ben experienced occurs for everyone who follows the Action Hero plan. Around that time, your body kicks into high gear, your hard work begins to pay off in noticeable changes in your physique and a sense of well-being, and you lose weight even though you've gained muscle. This is when you'll realize the program really will work for you, and you'll begin to feel like an Action Hero. If you can make it to the 3-week turnaround, you'll have a greater chance of continuing and accomplishing your personal fitness goals and setting yourself up for a lifetime of strength, health, and good looks.

Over time, you'll learn to regulate your body and diet so that you don't crave junk food and you actually enjoy your AH nutrition plan. You'll also understand how it's possible to follow the program, as I have, for years.

Are you beginning to see how the plan might work for you? It's not a crash course, but a long-term lifestyle change. Rest days are very important on the program. Overtraining or depleting your system, as you might have done in the past, is the last thing I want you to do.

Half of the Action Hero plan involves disciplining yourself in order to establish new habits. But the other half is about being provided with the right answers. You'll find them here. Most people who exercise with the idea of changing their physique think that more intense effort and unrealistic diets will get them to their goals sooner. They'll head as fast as they can down the wrong path until they burn out. It's like a plane de-

ACTION!

Action Hero: Josh Hartnett

Career accomplishments: MTV Movie Award for Best Breakthrough Performance in *Halloween H₂O: 20 Years Later.* Josh also appeared in the thriller *The Faculty* and the acclaimed indie flick *The Virgin Suicides.* He's starred in the feature films *Pearl Harbor, Othello, Black Hawk Down,* and *40 Days and 40 Nights.*

Physical goals: A more proportioned body with well-developed chest, shoulders, and arms.

Training program: Mostly superset workouts with little or no cardiovascular activity.

Results: He obtained his goal and developed more upper-body definition and muscle tone. What's more, Josh eventually developed an interest in the workouts (initially, he did not like weight lifting at all). He even called me up in Hawaii, where he was on location for *Pearl Harbor,* to work out, even though he wasn't scheduled to.

Josh is a nice guy from the Midwest. He's very calm, respectful, has a strong sense of family values, and has a great set of morals and ethics.

He had virtually no background in weight lifting, but he loved yoga, which gave him a great sense of his body and the know-how to involve his mind in the workouts. It was a breeze for me to explain about the Action Hero training system. In no time, he was doing flat-bench dumbbell presses with a pair of 50-pound dumbbells.

We accomplished a lot during the brief time we worked together, and as you can see in the love scene with Kate Beckinsale in *Pearl Harbor,* he truly can carry the title of "Action Hero"!

The gradual introduction to weight lifting helps a body avoid injuries to the muscles and joints and prepares it for the intense workouts for muscle development.

scending too quickly toward the landing strip. If it descends too quickly, it'll crash.

That's too extreme.

You want to take the middle road, tweaking your metabolism, raising your basal metabolic rate (see "Calculating Basal Metabolic Rate"), and slowly accumulating the small gains that add up to dramatic changes. The Action Hero program is about muscle gain and fat loss, and raising that metabolic rate which will ultimately lead to an athletic physique. You'll learn how to work with your body to achieve this until the program seems like second nature.

Finally, and perhaps most important, there's the notion of emotional detachment. You'll learn to look at the program as something you either do or don't do. There's no middle ground, no making excuses or justifying going off the plan.

That might sound harsh, but actually emotional detachment simplifies things greatly. You won't be tempted to cheat, because you'll have committed yourself to the plan. As the positive results start to manifest, they'll motivate you to stay with it.

A MAN WITHOUT A PLAN

Last year, one of my clients, a man named Tom Simes, e-mailed me because he needed to get fit. His doctor had told him, "Cut calories, and you'll be fine." So Tom went home and started cutting calories from his already inadequate nutrition program.

He stopped eating protein. But without this critical building block for muscle tissue, his body wasn't getting the nutrients it needed. Also, his metabolic rate dropped, because it wasn't activated by proper fat-burning exercise such as walking, hiking, or other low-impact activities. And he wasn't training with weights.

Tom lost weight all right, but the wrong kind, and he still felt far from his Action Hero goals.

We set up a sound nutrition plan for him, according to proper dietary guidelines, and *boom!* In a single month, he dropped roughly 12 pounds. He now maintains his diet, exercises more, and lives a much healthier lifestyle.

All the energy you expend fretting and thinking about what you're *supposed* to be doing can instead be put into simply doing it. You'll see that the more you cultivate this attitude, the easier the program becomes.

Why not give it a try? As long as you stay with it, I guarantee that it will work for you.

CALCULATING BASAL METABOLIC RATE

Use the formulas below to calculate your approximate basal metabolic rate (BMR). There are different formulas for men and women because men, as a rule, start out with more muscle mass than women and therefore burn more calories through their basal metabolism.

$$\text{Women: } 655 + (9.6 \times W) + (1.7 \times H) - (4.7 \times A) = BMR$$

$$\text{Men: } 66 + (13.7 \times W) + (5 \times H) - (6.8 \times A) = BMR$$

(W= Weight in kilograms, H = Height in centimeters, A = Age in years)

(To convert pounds to kilograms: divide weight in pounds by 2.2.)

(To convert inches to centimeters: multiply height in inches by 2.54.)

Digestion. Approximately 10 percent of the calories you take in are burned just processing the food you consume. For instance, if you consume 2,000 calories a day, you burn 200 of them by just digesting the food. In effect, eating helps you burn calories in the same way exercise does, just to a lesser extent.

Physical activity. Anywhere from 15 to 40 percent of your calorie burn comes from all of the various activities you perform throughout the day. Physical activity is the single most important component of caloric expenditure that you can control.

When people think of burning calories, they think of vigorous exercise, such as jogging or playing tennis. However, many people forget that all physical activity burns additional calories.

For instance, people who are taking the elevator instead of the stairs—but are getting up extra early to exercise in the hopes of burning extra calories—may be cheating themselves, because taking the stairs also burns calories. Even activities as simple as getting up to change the television channel instead of using the remote control burn calories.

Reminding yourself of those extra calories you burn during the simplest tasks may help you to invoke healthier lifestyle habits by simply taking advantage of your own mobility.

Self-Evaluation

FOR STAGE ONE

If you answer yes to all of the following questions, then you're ready to get on the path to becoming an Action Hero.

✔ Have I been training with weights or any other exercise equipment for less than 3 months, or not at all?

✔ Am I out of shape, either overweight or too skinny, but still relatively healthy (I have no joint, muscle, or organ problems and take only over-the-counter medication when I really need it)?

✔ Am I eager to make a radical change in my life that will make me strong and healthy, with a great-looking body?

✔ Am I willing to believe, trust, and follow the instructions in this book to a T?

✔ Will nothing stop me, even when I get frustrated, tired, hungry, and irritated at times?

FOR STAGE TWO

If you answer yes to all of the following questions, then you're ready for Stage Two of the Action Hero training system.

✔ Have I been training for more than a year off and on, and have I reached a certain understanding of training with weights?

✔ Am I still bothered by some excess fat, and do I want to get lean and muscular, or do I want to put on some serious muscle?

✔ Even though I have a basic understanding of training, am I still looking for guidance to get it down once and for all?

FOR STAGE THREE

If you answer yes to the following questions, then you can confidently throw yourself into Stage Three. You're ready to swim with the big fish. But still read through Stage One and Stage Two—I'm sure you'll find something interesting that you didn't know before.

✓ Have I been training for multiple years, and have I reached a certain level of development in my physique?

✓ Do I know my personal limits—that is, how much weight I can lift with virtually every exercise or machine in my gym?

✓ Have I reached a plateau in my workouts, and am I having trouble pushing through it to reach new heights in my strength, muscle tone, and muscle definition?

Setting Goals

Besides setting the *big* goal to become an Action Hero, with all the benefits and satisfaction that implies, you must begin to change your lifestyle on other fronts as well. You can do this by setting smaller minigoals that will lead you to the ultimate one.

Here's a sample list of goals you might consider in your pursuit of "getting there."

1. Make the ultimate promise to yourself and *only* to yourself that you're going to follow the guidelines in this book.

2. Organize your life so that you'll be able to follow the Action Hero training system—specifically, the nutrition part. Clear out all the junk food from your home and replace it with the nutritious components you'll need to stay on course. These include vegetables, lean meat, eggs, oatmeal, and fresh bottled water.

3. Update your membership at your local gym and start making time in your already hectic schedule to work out. It might mean that you give up a couple of nights lounging in front of the TV. You'll soon realize that it was one of the best things you've ever done.

4. If you already visit the gym regularly, sit down and rethink your current workout program and alter it based on the guidelines in this book.

5. If you have a close friend who's in the same position as you, invite him or her to buddy up with you as you follow the path to an Action Hero physique.

6. Dig up a picture of yourself from an era when you were in good shape—your college football days or high school wrestling team years—and stick it on your refrigerator or bathroom mirror. Or display some item of clothing you've had for years and don't fit into anymore. Use these objects to motivate you to stay focused on the big goal.

7. When you begin, follow the plan for 3 weeks without any deviations or delays. No excuses or justifications for abandoning it once you've started. Give it 3 solid weeks of your best effort.

8. Make a habit of planning ahead. For instance, prepare a Jørgy-style Montiff shake the night before and bring it to work with you in a small cooler. That way, if you're stuck in the car or at the office, you can reach for a quick, healthy meal instead of running to the vending machine.

9. Once you have committed to every detail of the Action Hero lifestyle, think of it as a goal for a lifetime. An Action Hero physique is something that you'll want to have forever, and it's possible by following the plan every day for the rest of your life.

ACTION!

Action Hero: Bridget Moynahan

Career accomplishments: Besides her role in *Coyote Ugly,* Bridget has appeared in *Whipped, Serendipity, Sum of All Fears, The Recruit,* and *I, Robot.*

Physical goals: Rock-hard abs and upper-body strength to enable her to hang and do chinups from metal pipes in the movie *Coyote Ugly.*

Training program: For this particular task, she started with knee pushups and worked up to regular pushups. From supported chinups, she advanced to regular chinups in combination with regular back, chest, leg, shoulder, and arm exercises. I recommended a limited amount of aerobic activity, because Bridget had a low percentage of body fat to begin with.

Results: Bridget got ripped, rock-hard, and chiseled abs in 2 weeks (the movie's producer didn't believe it was possible).

At first, I didn't meet with Bridget, because three women from the cast were already working out with me, and though they already looked really sculpted, they needed me the most. But Bridget kept calling the producer and finally got the okay to work out with me. It was a delight to work with her. Even though she can be a little intimidating, she was always friendly, respectful, and ready to crack a joke.

I soon found out that Bridget was a hard worker who took not only her acting seriously but everything around it as well: workouts, auditions, dieting, even punctuality. Everything had to be at its best. She is the ideal female Action Hero.

Usually, I took Bridget through a superset workout. For instance: back and triceps followed by another round of back and triceps, but with a different combination of exercises. Then rear delts and biceps, and we'd finish off with an isolation back exercise, such as the Lat Flex, combined with a few more biceps sets.

If you haven't seen Bridget in one of the many magazines or movies she's appeared in, go to a Web site that mentions her and check her out for yourself.

Hard and intense abdominal workouts are a necessary part of the Action Hero routine.

THE ACTION HERO
NUTRITION PLAN

4

FUEL FOR THE BODY

THINK OF A SPORTS CAR. If you want it to move fast and live up to your expectations, you must give it the right fuel and follow the instructions in the owner's manual. The car will then deliver top performance at cruising speed and accelerate with no effort.

The same concept applies to your body. If you eat the right food, you'll perform the way your body was designed, and beyond.

Let's take the sports car analogy one step further. If you step hard on the gas pedal every time you drive, never change the oil, and never wash or wax your shiny new car, after a few years it will look and run like a beater destined for the junkyard.

Now picture this: You own a sports car, and you love it dearly. You drive it sensibly, and occasionally you cruise the freeway at 100 miles an hour. Every 3,000 miles you change the oil, and you spend weekends washing and waxing this beauty. Your car can take its place with those classic Porsches and Ferraris that look like new and sound as if they just rolled off the factory line.

Naturally, one day your car will quit working, but it will have performed optimally all its life, with few mechanical problems.

Likewise, people who know how to take care of themselves—through a healthy diet, exercise, and rest—will live longer, healthier, more productive lives. It's not that complicated. Even if your car is dirty and it hasn't had an oil and lube job in a while, it can be repaired. So, too, can your body. It's never too late to change your lifestyle.

"I'm a WWII U.S. Army Infantry veteran and have been working out with Jørgen for the last 6 years," says POM Wonderful executive Berton Steir, 79, a longtime client of mine. "As a result, I'm in better condition now than I was 20 years ago. Whether it's one-on-one in the gym or by his written instructions when I'm traveling, I know that I can always maintain my present condition for years to come. Mark these words: 'It's never too late to get back into shape.'"

The Nutrition Equation

When we talk about diet, we're not talking about starving yourself or eating only bland foods. Diets are designed in harmony with what the body needs internally. When you adjust your diet so that it delivers sound nutrients to your body, your body begins to balance itself and optimize the functionality of all organs, including the skin. It ultimately will lead to a well-proportioned physique. I know people who live healthy lifestyles and who don't work out with any real intensity, and they're tall and slender with no excess body fat. Their diets consist of fruits, grains and other complex carbohydrates, along with fish or other low-fat meat. How you look, or more important, *feel*, really depends on whether you treat yourself to a healthy lifestyle.

The problem with living an unhealthy lifestyle or even an incomplete one is that bad habits breed more bad habits. You come to accept this way of living as normal (see "Follow the Guidelines" on page 5). By the age of 30, this "normal" lifestyle can lead to joint pains, high blood pressure, organ failure, a shortened life—you name it.

On the other hand, when your body receives food in the right combination of protein, carbohydrates, fat, vitamins, and minerals, it becomes a fat-burning, calorie-consuming machine that can rebuild itself after work and exercise.

Every food item has its purpose. You don't want to live solely on meals designed to tickle your tastebuds. Foods such as chips, pasta with cream sauce, pizza, and hamburgers—you know the list—typically are high in fat and glucose (sugar). Also, the total caloric count is too high for our bodies to assimilate.

These foods lack essential nutrients such as protein, complex carbohydrates, vitamins, and minerals.

When people are gaining weight, they simply have to go on a diet that delivers just the right amount of calories. No more, no less. This requires a lifestyle change, eating fewer calories than you burn. Once you've reached your goal, then and only then should you rethink your diet.

But just cutting calories isn't the way to go, unless you want to lose your muscle tissue, and quickly. Here's why: If you live on a low-calorie, unbalanced diet, you end up eating unhealthy food with little or no nutritional value, and you deprive your body of the nutrients it needs to maintain muscles, bones, and organs. As a result, your body becomes less efficient and burns fewer calories (see "A Man without a Plan" on page 26).

If you're of the mindset that you can live an entire life without a controlled nutrition program, think again. Over time, you *will* gain weight, which is really the sign of overconsumption of food and a body that's ready to give up and give out. Many of you probably have already experienced diets. You'll go on a "weight-loss" program, then later go back to your old ways (eating more calories than you burn). Slowly, but ultimately, you begin to gain weight.

But change your entire lifestyle—keeping your body weight in check and feeding your body the appropriate amount of nutrients—and there *will* be room to eat foods that are bad for the body, but taste wonderful. But let's not get ahead of ourselves.

As a rule: If something tastes good, it's probably not good for your body. If something tastes bland, it's probably not high in calories, high in fat, high in sugar, or high in sodium. As a rule, it'll be better for your body.

Say Adiós to Old Habits

For many individuals, food has become a form of comfort. They've learned to use it to alleviate something that's missing emotionally. For instance, if you're depressed, you might eat comfort foods that aren't particularly healthy. Then, when depression begins to linger, your unhealthy eating habits become a pattern. Once the pattern sets in, even when the depression is gone, both the body and mind crave or depend upon the wrong kinds of food.

Then there's the entertainment factor. "Let's meet for dinner"; "Let's go to the ballpark and eat hot dogs, burgers, and fries." Every street corner has a fast-food restaurant. It's insane!

These days, food must have extraordinary taste in order for most people to enjoy eating. All too often, a broiled chicken breast doesn't appeal to our tastebuds, whereas rotisserie chicken baked in its own fat and added butter—well, you get the picture.

Fat, sugar, salt—and lots of them—are the main tastemakers in the average American's diet, and these undermine the nutritional value of a balanced, healthy diet. Processed foods such as chips, ice cream, and packaged snacks are the worst in this respect.

Food should be considered what it truly is: fuel to nourish your body and mind (the mind, by the way, is a valid part of the body). Food

MEAL TIPS

• Start the day with high carbohydrates and taper it down as the day progresses. Divide your carbohydrates into 70 percent complex carbs and 30 percent simple carbs.

• Keep your protein intake moderate and consistent and your fat low and consistent throughout the day.

• Most of your calories should be consumed at breakfast and lunch. Choose food with fewer calories and make the portions smaller for dinner.

• Drink at least ½ gallon (about eight glasses) of pure water every day. Start by drinking a large glass of pure water with every meal, including snacks. I even drink a large glass of water when I wake up in the morning.

• Don't cheat on your diet during the week (Monday through Friday). I cannot stress this enough.

• Cut down on coffee (one strong cup in the morning or a double espresso), limit diet sodas to two a day, and eliminate smoking or cut back to five or fewer cigarettes a day.

• Keep your alcohol consumption to a minimum. No more than three glasses of wine or three beers per week.

• Never miss a meal.

• Avoid all added fat such as butter, lard, and fatty meat.

• Avoid all simple sugars such as refined white sugar, candies, and juices.

• Include 1 to 3 teaspoons of olive oil per day as a valid part of your diet. Put it in your egg whites, shakes, salads, or vegetables.

• Use dressings sparingly, and only the fat-free kind. Otherwise, use vinegar.

• Go easy on juices and fruit.

replaces valuable nutrients and supplies building blocks to repair used and damaged cells. It can't solve your emotional problems, and it shouldn't be confused with entertainment.

The dietary guidelines outlined in this book might seem a little too structured at first: no alcohol, no butter when cooking, and a lot more rules. What's more, the results of these dietary changes won't be apparent for a few weeks.

Let me repeat: *The results of these changes won't be apparent for a few weeks.*

At first you'll feel as if you're sacrificing a lot. But after a few weeks, you'll start to notice more strength, endurance, muscle—and less fat. You'll have more energy during your workouts, a happier outlook on life, and a deeper appreciation of your new lifestyle.

The true objective of any diet or plan you commit yourself to is to

A WORD OR TWO ABOUT WATER

People still don't drink enough water. Maybe these simple facts will get your attention.

• About 75 percent of all Americans are chronically dehydrated.

• For 37 percent of Americans, the thirst mechanism is so weak that it's often mistaken for hunger.

• Even mild dehydration will slow down one's metabolism by as much as 3 percent.

• One glass of water will shut down midnight hunger pangs for nearly 100 percent of dieters, according to a University of Washington study.

• Lack of water is the number-one trigger of daytime fatigue.

• Preliminary research indicates that eight to 10 glasses of water a day could significantly ease back and joint pain for up to 80 percent of sufferers.

• A mere 2 percent drop in body water can trigger short-term memory loss, trouble with basic math, and difficulty focusing on the computer screen or a printed page.

• Drinking five glasses of water daily decreases the risk of colon cancer by 45 percent.

make improvements. Don't fixate on the end result. Once you've decided to make this commitment, to live the life of an Action Hero, don't think about the end results. Instead, take it one day at a time. Even small improvements over your previous lifestyle are crucial to meeting your goals.

For instance, simply replacing your soda consumption with water will dramatically improve how you replenish your muscles, which consist of 90 percent water—*not* soda. Water is an important building block and cleanser for the body. Soda, on the other hand, has too much sugar, chemicals, and caffeine. The sugar is converted into fat, and caffeine is a diuretic that strips your body of water and essential micronutrients such as vitamins and minerals.

Naturally, you can't expect to make all these dietary changes from day one. Your rewards—which will include better sleep and improved physical condition (externally as well as internally)—will come in time.

Of course, it's up to you whether you stick to the plan, so don't justify and rationalize. Once you start making excuses, you'll soon be back to your old habits. Deviations will result in delay or even failure. Stick to the plan (see "Plan Ahead" on page 77).

And if you find yourself in that situation at a restaurant with people eating unhealthy food—creamy pasta dishes, pizza, steak and french fries, lamb chops with gravy, buttered vegetables, desserts—just say no (see "Restaurant Strategies" on page 60). It's not easy, I realize. But it *is* that simple. If you can muster that kind of discipline and willpower, you can conquer anything.

Never Deprive Yourself; Instead, Compromise

In general, we don't like to deprive ourselves of rich food. That's fine if you're within 10 pounds of your optimal body weight and you only eat bad calories every once in a while. Sure, you might get a little instant gratification from the sugar and fat, but you'll also feel sluggish, bloated, and unable to do any athletic activity for about 3 hours.

I know it's hard to start cutting good-tasting food from your diet. But if you want to feel and look like an Action Hero, you must cut most, if not all, of the "bad" food. Keep in mind, though, that when you've reached your fitness goals in record time, you can reintroduce some of the treats you had to cut out at the beginning. But you'll do this rationally, adding certain kinds of food, at certain times of the day, in certain amounts.

In other words, when you decide to go overboard, once you have reached your goal, you can. But you'll do it sensibly by choosing relatively nutritious "junk" food such as gourmet pizza, wholesome burgers, one ice cream cone, French toast, steak and wild rice, Caesar salad with chicken, pasta Bolognese with meatballs, and so on. Just avoid fried foods, high-fat meats, pastries, and chocolate candy bars, which contain virtually no nutritional value.

For the most part, I live on egg whites (cooked any style); lean, skinless chicken breasts with herbs and spices; lean steak; sometimes fish; oatmeal; vegetables; fruit; rice; a Montiff meal-replacement supplement; and water (see "Fit Forever: My Weekly Action Hero Lifestyle" on page 70). But I also love an occasional slice of pizza, hamburgers, and ice cream. Typically on weekends, I'll allow myself some of these in moderation, so that I don't feel deprived, which is why most people resist restricted-calorie diets.

Let me spell it out for you: You *will not* have the body of an Action Hero if junk food and other high-calorie food items make up the bulk of your diet.

How to Change Your Eating Habits

What you must first do is find out what you're actually eating day by day, week by week, and month by month. Write everything down, from the water you drink to the smallest snack you buy at a vending machine. Remember to include even healthy food such as fruits and vegetables, and definitely all the food you eat at any restaurant, from fast food to fine dining. In short, *everything*. Then figure out how many calories you've actually eaten. You can easily go to any bookstore and purchase a calorie-counter booklet, which will give you all the calorie numbers you need. You'll be amazed at how much of what you currently eat is actually garbage.

Then we can get to work stripping your current daily food plan of all the unnecessary stuff and replacing it with food that will work for you—not against you. To make this process easier, I've designed for you a nutritionally sound way of living, based on your height and your Action Hero weight goal. Granted, in the beginning you might feel as though this lifestyle just isn't working. Every now and then, you might waver or lose focus. I can almost guarantee, however, that these doubts

LET THE GOOD GUYS TAKE CHARGE

Let's assume you've decided to commit yourself to the Action Hero training system. The first 3 weeks will be the most challenging, because there's no instant gratification with this plan. You will, however, notice improvements in your energy and performance levels during these crucial weeks of your workouts.

The toughest tests will come when you're in social settings, or when you're mentally tired or stressed. As long as you can identify these vulnerable times and take charge, you'll be able to persevere. Keep reminding yourself that the weight is coming off and the muscle is coming on. Soon enough, you'll get leaner, with more tone and more muscularity. Notice how people start complimenting you on your appearance. You'll begin to feel a well-deserved sense of accomplishment, and that will help you stay motivated.

I tell my son that the bad guys are those foods that make him tired and unhealthy, and the good guys are those foods that want to beat up the bad guys. It works for him. Actually, it works for me, too. Fortunately, I was born with a strong sense of discipline. As I learned more about what unhealthy foods could do to a person, I realized I'd become fat and unhealthy if I wasn't disciplined. That knowledge was enough to keep me motivated. Also, I didn't think in terms of following a restricted "diet." Instead, I thought about how privileged I was to have gained an understanding of a healthy way of living.

will disappear after the first 3 weeks, or at, as I like to call it, the 3-week turnaround.

My program is best viewed as a process with distinctive workouts. The first stage is the 3-week turnaround. After 3 weeks on the Action Hero program, positive changes will start to surface: more endurance, a happier and more vital life, weight loss, increased strength, even the signs of a more muscular body, and better cardiovascular output. Don't expect too many changes until then. But in order for this program to work, you must plan ahead and execute.

Also, don't forget to support this program with vitamins and supplements (see chapter 6), water, and rest.

Naturally, there will be temptations, appetite surges, even excuses to break your strategy. For instance, if you're the type who eats too much refined sugar, and all of a sudden you switch to fruits only, your body might resist and you'll feel some withdrawal symptoms.

You might also be plagued by increased appetite, which shouldn't be confused with real hunger. This could be caused by the sudden drop in calories. There's no need to worry, though, because I've already calculated the calorie intake of your Action Hero diet, supplying you with a sufficient amount of protein, carbohydrates, and fats to answer your body's demands. Soon enough, all the elements of this system will kick in, and the new you will begin to emerge. Once you've cruised through that first 3-week period, you will come to understand what it truly means to be an Action Hero.

The Give and Take of Losing Fat, Gaining Muscle

During the first few weeks of your Action Hero plan, you'll lose weight right off the bat. Your pants will become looser around your waist, and you'll start to notice definition in your arms. However, after a few more weeks, your weight loss will taper off and might even come to a complete stop.

Don't panic.

This is the time your body starts to respond to the workouts and your sensible nutrition program.

When you work out hard with weights, your muscle tissue breaks down from the stress. However, a combination of proper nutrition and rest between workouts helps your muscles repair themselves. During this rebuilding process, they become bigger and stronger. In reality, you haven't stopped losing fat weight, but your muscle mass has increased, and because muscle weighs more than fat, your scale won't register the loss. For instance, if you lose 3 pounds of fat weight and gain an incredible 3 pounds of muscle, the scale won't move, but you're still accomplishing your goal. It's important to keep this in mind when you get discouraged. Instead, you should get motivated. It's a step forward.

Once your muscle growth hits a possible, temporary plateau, the scale will start to move down again. You want to make sure, though, that you don't lose the pounds too quickly. If you do, then you're training too hard or eating too little, or a combination of the two, and you'll lose that hard-earned muscle tissue through lack of nutrients and overtraining.

If anything, you might have to back off from the aerobic activity or increase your calories a bit, or both, to adjust to your increased physical needs. Remember: In simplified form, more protein equals more building and rebuilding blocks for muscle tissue; more carbohydrates equals more energy. In the end, your body will find its core weight.

Spiral Up, Spiral Down

This is probably the easiest way to explain what happens when you gain weight, as in getting fat and unhealthy. I describe it as a negative spiral-up, spiral-down syndrome.

Often, when you gain 15 pounds or more, you don't even notice the difference until it's too late. But in order to gain 15 pounds of fat or more, you must have eaten a lot of extra calories for an extended period of time, and your body has gradually become less efficient.

As you get heavier, you get less and less active. This in turns causes you to gain even more weight. Once you come to the realization that you're overweight, most of you will try to cut back on what you eat, which decreases the calories from an already low-quality-food diet. As a result, your bodily functions slow down and certain organs decrease their functionality. As you get heavier, your body, joints, tendons, and ligaments get taxed more dramatically. You're less able to maintain your muscle tone and mass to uphold your increasingly heavier body. Your muscles in turn become too weakened even for the occasional weekend sporting event.

Soon enough you're 25 or even 30 pounds overweight. Your cholesterol and blood pressure have increased, your heart's working overtime, and your metabolic rate has diminished dramatically. And yet, some of you continue to eat and eat and eat. You may even say to yourself, "Who cares if I gain another pound?"

It's like when someone is up to his neck in credit card debt and figures, "Who cares if I charge another $100? I can't pay my balance anyway."

Personally, I have never had credit card debt, and I have never been more than 10 pounds over my AH goal weight. Simply put, I don't want to deal with the stress and hardship of either situation.

But, as you optimize the actual calories that you eat, your body starts to burn fat more efficiently. As a result, your body starts to work more efficiently with real nutrients. Think of your body as a campfire that needs good burning material to stay alive. A dry piece of wood—not too big, not too small—will fuel the fire, whereas a piece of plastic will incinerate in a heartbeat and even diminish the fury of the fire.

The bad lifestyle is a negative spiral up/down. The spiral up represents increased weight, increased blood pressure, and increased risk of major illnesses such as heart disease and diabetes. The spiral down represents a lower metabolic rate, decreased muscle tone, a decreased sex drive, and lower productivity in the workplace.

BAD LIFESTYLE DOUBLE SPIRAL

INCREASED WEIGHT
INCREASED BLOOD PRESSURE
INCREASED RISK OF
MAJOR ILLNESS SUCH AS
HEART DISEASE, DIABETES, ETC.

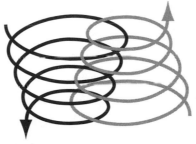

LOWER METABOLIC RATE
DECREASED MUSCLE TONE
DECREASED SEX DRIVE
LOWER PRODUCTIVITY
IN THE WORKPLACE

The Action Hero lifestyle is a positive spiral up/down. The spiral up represents increased health, increased strength of muscular structure as well as bodily organs, increased stamina and endurance on all levels, and an increased sense of well-being. The spiral down represents lower body weight, lower blood pressure (in most cases), and less body fat while experiencing more muscularity.

ACTION HERO LIFESTYLE DOUBLE SPIRAL

INCREASED HEALTH
INCREASED STRENGTH
OF MUSCULAR STRUCTURE
AS WELL AS BODILY ORGANS
INCREASED STAMINA AND ENDURANCE
ON ALL LEVELS
INCREASED SENSE OF WELL-BEING

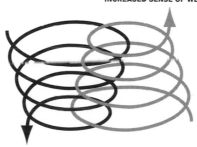

LOWER BODY WEIGHT
LOWER BLOOD PRESSURE
LESS BODY FAT
WHILE EXPERIENCING
MORE MUSCULARITY

The Truth about Weight Loss

A lot of people think they're overweight because they don't have time to exercise properly, what with work, family, and everything. There's always time to exercise. Imagine where your work and family would be if you died suddenly of a heart attack because you never found the time to exercise. To stay well-conditioned takes only about 3 hours a week, once you have reached your Action Hero weight goal.

But this isn't the real reason people are overweight. The fact is, most people still believe that as long as they do a little (or even a lot) of car-

QUALITY-OF-LIFE COMPARISON

Now that we've examined the effects of living each of these lifestyles, let's see what you can expect your quality of life to be like through each decade.

THE AVERAGE AMERICAN LIFESTYLE

• Twenties—No significant difference between someone who lives in accordance with the average American lifestyle or the AH lifestyle. However, the athlete who eats well, exercises, and rests enough will always have the edge.

• Thirties—This is the time that the average American lifestyle will take its toll. It will manifest itself in more sluggish behavior, the unwanted love handles, more injuries at work or play, and longer recovery time from injuries.

• Forties—You often hear it said: "I'm too old for that!" or "My cholesterol and blood pressure are way too high, and I'm taking meds for it." The cumulative effects of years of bad habits are taking their toll on the body in the form of even more injuries. Most 40-year-olds develop a significant belly and are 40 pounds over their projected Action Hero weight goal.

• Fifties—By the time the average American has reached age 50, it's over as far as sports are concerned. Years of bad diet have taken their toll; the organs don't work as well as they once did. It's sad.

• Sixties and beyond—I haven't seen too many average Americans at this age living life to its fullest, but it's definitely possible. Unfortunately, few men and women in their sixties take the necessary steps to maintain a healthy lifestyle.

diovascular activity, they can eat pretty much what they want without getting fat and still become lean.

Sure, with cardiovascular activity your overall physical condition might improve, but you'll still be carrying around extra weight. Also, as you age, your metabolism slows down, and before you know it, you've gained extra weight.

Yet another wrong idea: avoiding carbohydrates altogether. Not all carbs are created equal. I'm still amazed that people will avoid nutritious *complex* carbohydrates such as rice, bread, and certain cereals, but don't think twice about consuming *simple* carbs such as sugar—which, by the

THE ACTION HERO LIFESTYLE

• Twenties—No significant difference between the average American lifestyle and the Action Hero lifestyle.

• Thirties—The man who started his AH lifestyle in his twenties will be in optimal health in his thirties if there are no major genetic problems. He will bounce back quickly after the rare cold or flu, and he'll have no problem with his blood pressure or cholesterol. He will still be able to run back and forth on the basketball court and play tennis or ice hockey.

• Forties—He may have to stretch a little more before every sporting event, but a 40-year-old man on the AH program will have the appearance of a man in his thirties.

• Fifties and sixties—The AH man is still working out, still playing on the court, still having fun. Expressions are now: "I feel great; it feels like I'm still in my forties!" or "I have a great outlook on life and I still love to travel!"

• Seventies—I have one 78-year-old client who works 5 days a week in the office and works out in the gym two or three times a week. It has made him young again (he started the AH lifestyle at 72). No ailment, no medication. He's in tip-top condition.

CONCLUSION? You not only will potentially live longer than you would have without the AH lifestyle, but also the quality *throughout* your life will be far superior.

way, is everywhere: in sodas, snacks, even so-called "health bars" (see "All Calories Are Not Created Equal" on page 14).

Most people think sugar is better than complex carbs because their bodies will burn it right away. It's true that your body will use the sugar immediately, but not all of it. If there's too much sugar, the remainder gets stored as fat.

On the other hand, complex carbohydrates in moderate portions are converted into glycogen and stored in the muscles and liver. From there, the glycogen is easily converted into energy for all kinds of bodily functions, including muscle contractions and brain activity.

True Confessions: Tell It to Your Log

You'll make progress toward your fitness goals faster if you maintain a diet log. A log is simply a small notebook that you carry around with you. Every time you put something in your mouth to eat or drink, write down the time, item, and amount. Also write down the time slots during the day that you're free for a workout. Keep your log for 2 weeks.

Next, figure out how many calories you consume per day. You can do this by reading the nutrition labels on the food, and by purchasing a pocket calorie counter that lists food items alphabetically and provides the caloric information for each one. It won't take you long to memorize the calories in your favorite foods, especially if you're writing the amount down every time.

Of course, because everyone's metabolism is different, daily caloric intake will vary from person to person. For some, 1,500 calories will get them through a day, while others require about 2,500 calories. I've simplified this process by providing you with three diet plans based on your height and Action Hero weight goal.

Now you can start thinking about your own nutrition program, according to the AH diet method—no sugar or alcohol, keep the fat down and the protein up. Your most important objective is to make sure you get an adequate amount of protein because it's the building block and regulator of your muscles, organs, and brain.

It's important that the protein is consumed in equal portions throughout the day to maintain a positive nitrogen balance (the difference between the amount of nitrogen taken into the body and the amount excreted or lost).

This balance between nitrogen input and output indicates whether you're getting an adequate amount of protein, which in turn will determine whether you build muscle or lose it. The remainder of your diet should consist of calories divided between carbohydrates (70 percent complex, 30 percent simple) and predominantly unsaturated fat. Fat shouldn't make up more than 30 percent of anyone's total caloric intake.

When I look over logs from my aspiring Action Heroes, I always ask them whether they were surprised by the sort of foods they were eating and how many calories they contained. When they begin paying attention to what and how much they eat, they become aware of how different foods affect their physical and emotional well-being.

First I recommend that they replace all the bad food with good. For example, if for breakfast you typically eat a bowl of cereal with 2% milk and three scrambled eggs with bacon, you can easily change that to shredded wheat with fat-free milk and four egg whites. (Don't even start with me about turkey bacon. It's a no-no.) You'll notice that I haven't really dropped any volume or amount of food, but I've replaced the stuff that's bad for you with stuff that's good, and we've cut the amount of calories by more than half.

Here's another example: Hidden fat is in lots of different food, but particularly packaged meals and snacks. Even when a product is described as low-fat, it's not. For example, most people assume that the "99% fat-free" printed on a yogurt container means only 1 percent of the total calories is derived from fat.

Wrong.

Look instead at where it tells you about calories per serving versus fat per serving: under "Amount per Serving" in the Nutrition Facts label.

Calories: 170

Calories from fat: 15

Read the label again, and you'll see that it says 170 calories and 1.5 grams of fat. Do your math: 1.5 *grams* of fat is not 1 percent of 170 *calories*. It's like comparing apples and pears. Why? Because 1.5 grams of fat equals roughly 15 calories (1 gram of fat equals 9 calories), and 15 of 170 calories equals almost 10 percent fat.

Be smart. Do your homework.

THE DEADLY WHITE STUFF

Based on its molecular structure, sugar falls in the category of simple carbohydrates. It's highly refined and therefore lacking in good things like fiber, vitamins, minerals, and other nutrients. This makes it not only less nutritious than complex carbohydrates such as brown rice and whole wheat bread, but also less filling.

What's more, your body tends to digest sugar more quickly than it does complex carbs, and this messes with your insulin levels to give you the infamous sugar high followed by a slump. Invariably, you set up a cycle where you end up craving more sugar. Sound like a drug? As far as your body is concerned, it is. Sugar also has been linked to problems such as high cholesterol, an overabundance of fat in the bloodstream, and mineral deficiencies that can lead to heart disease or diabetes.

So do yourself a favor and start stripping away unnecessary sugar from your diet. By this I mean sugar in your coffee, sweet stuff on your toast, candy bars, cookies, fat-free snacks, breath mints (nothing but empty calories in those), even those highly advertised meal replacement bars. Also eliminate most of your sodas, juices, sports drinks, and smoothies; they're loaded with sugar. One can of soda contains the equivalent of 12 cubes of pure, white, refined sugar, most of which will be turned into fat—when it's not rotting your teeth. (Don't worry; I'm not a hard-core health nut, and I won't deny you a little pleasure such as occasional diet sodas. But that's it.)

Replace these items with healthy substitutes—such as apples, papaya, mangos, grapes, or blueberries—whose calories your body will use to good purpose. Don't forget that sugar, when it's not used by the body right away, is converted into fat and stored somewhere in the body.

But let's stay focused on what we have to do, and that's strip the fat from your diet. Cut the fried food—and yes, that includes potato chips, whether they're plain, flavored, or even baked. Eliminate salami, fast-food-style hamburgers, whole-egg omelets, and any chicken that still has the skin on it. Avoid anything that has a fat content higher than the protein content. To figure that out, make sure that you convert the grams into calories, because although 4 grams of fat may seem like less than 8 grams of protein, it's not. Four grams of fat equates to 36 calories, and 8 grams of protein equates to 32 calories! One gram of fat equates to 9 calories, 1 gram of protein equates to 4 calories, and 1 gram of carbohydrates, 4 calories. Read the labels on the food you buy, and don't be fooled anymore by descriptions such as "extra lean."

Naturally, anything that's prepared with fat tastes better. But know this: When you're on the Action Hero plan, your tastebuds are much more sensitive—or they will be after you've cleaned all the bad stuff out of your system. You'll even get to the point where a piece of fruit will taste like candy.

Ultimately, these changes not only will lead to a dramatically reduced sugar and fat intake, but they'll increase protein and complex carbs while reducing your overall caloric intake by 30 to 40 percent. However, you'll notice that, once you've cut the sugar and fat from your diet, not much food is left to list in your daily log. Stay with me, and I'll show you how to fill those empty spaces with nutritious and tasty food items.

Rethinking Your Meals

For those of you who don't eat breakfast, get over yourselves. Breakfast really is the most important meal of the day, so make sure you work it into your daily routine. And to keep you going until lunch, eat a piece of fruit (preferably one with a low glycemic index) or some kind of complex carbohydrate such as pretzels or maybe (maybe!) a small 150-calorie granola bar in between breakfast and lunch.

When it comes to lunch, most people don't know how to prepare for it and instead eat one of those "gourmet" frozen dinners or stop at fast-food restaurants. Their only consideration is that the meal should tickle their tastebuds. Businesspeople in particular like to eat off the menu at restaurants. A restaurant meal typically accounts for 700 to 800 calories, or even more, most of which are predominantly from fat, and that's not even including an appetizer and dessert.

Or maybe you're the type who munches on high-sugar, high-calorie granola bars or other snacks that don't deliver valuable nutrients. Then to make matters worse, you'll reach for a cookie and coffee or chips and soda in the afternoon to stay alert.

If you're serious about creating an Action Hero physique, you're going to have to let go of these bad habits and emotional attachments to food. Otherwise, you're doomed to fail. Forever!

As you scour your log for bad habits, look for things like the insane variety of snacks you go through in a day, the quick lunch at a fast-food restaurant, the sushi dinners with friends, or the late-night dinner with your wife.

GLYCEMIC INDEX

This is a rating system that indicates the different speed with which carbohydrates are processed into glucose by the body. In general, complex carbs are broken down more slowly, providing a moderate infusion of glucose for steady energy. Refined, simple carbs usually are absorbed quickly, causing energy-disturbing fluctuations of glucose.

Low-glycemic foods: fructose, soybeans, sweet potatoes, yams, apples (especially Golden Delicious), oranges, whole wheat products, brown rice, oats, and buckwheat pancakes

High-glycemic foods: honey, glucose, carrots, mashed potato, bananas, raisins, dried fruits, white rice, white bread, white spaghetti, and white flour pancakes

Dinner, by the way, is where most people go wrong. Let me make this clear: You must eat most of your calories before 2:00 P.M. Yes, it's true, your social life might suffer a little bit. But these are the sacrifices you must make if you want an Action Hero body.

When I glance over a person's log, usually one of the first things I notice is that there's not enough protein in the diet. Instead, there's an overabundance of fat and carbs such as muffins, bagels, and cereals high in sugar for breakfast; a sandwich with meat and mayonnaise and protein or granola bars for lunch; and pasta, rice, or potatoes and high-fat meats—prepared with butter and olive oil, of course—for dinner.

On average, a man with a moderately intensive workout regimen will need at least 80 grams of protein each day. To picture how that translates into food, 100 grams of protein amounts to about six egg whites, a turkey sandwich, a protein shake or protein bar, and a large piece of lean fish.

Let's say that you're trying to lose those last 10 extra pounds. Your caloric intake is calculated at 2,000 calories, and you burn a respectable 2,300 calories a day. You've nailed it! Those 300 calories will be burned off from your stored fat.

But let's also say that you get this craving for a favorite midafternoon snack or an ice cream cone after dinner while watching TV. Each of these "snacks" amounts to more than 300 calories. Some are more than 500 calories. In the brief time it takes you to eat a small bowl of ice cream, your caloric intake for that day has gone from a deficit to a surplus, meaning you're eating more calories than your body actually burns.

And then you wonder why you're not getting leaner.

All I'm saying is that the difference between your old form and an Action Hero physique might be just a few calories. It's a numbers game: If you eat 1 calorie less than you burn, you'll get leaner. If you eat 1 calorie more than you burn, you'll get fatter.

Enough said. Stay on course. Don't deviate. Don't delay.

ACTION!

Action Hero: Jerry O'Connell

Career accomplishments: Jerry began acting at the age of 11. His first screen role was in *Stand by Me.* He's made numerous films, television features, and miniseries, including *Crossing Jordan, Romeo Fire, Jerry Maguire, Mission to Mars, and Kangaroo Jack.*

Physical goals: To get him in tip-top shape for *Kangaroo Jack,* including muscular arms and shoulders and the much-admired six-pack.

Training program: Heavy weight lifting in accordance with the Action Hero training system, Stages Two and Three. Aerobic activity, such as walking on an inclined treadmill, or cardiovascular activity like running along Sunset Strip on nonworkout days.

Results: The producer was satisfied, Jerry O'Connell was satisfied, and I was satisfied.

When Jerry came to me, I was delighted to note that he was in good condition and that he worked out quite often. So, we began doing supersets right away, and even a giant circuit set, including racing on the stationary bike for 2-minute intervals.

Although Jerry was in good shape, I thought he needed some adjustments in his nutrition program. The grueling entertainment schedule was affecting his caloric intake: little or no breakfast, incomplete meals, and too much to eat for dinner.

It took a little while for Jerry to get used to the diet, because he didn't even own a microwave to heat up his oatmeal, let alone a pan, cooking spray, and eggs! Soon after we talked about it, he came to the gym one morning telling me proudly that he'd made oatmeal and eggs. I always say, "Where there's a will, there's a way!"

Even now, Jerry is a strong believer in the Action Hero lifestyle. Check him out on the TV program *Crossing Jordan* and judge for yourself.

Weight lifting in conjunction with cardio intervals on the stationary bike (or pushing The Cart) can help you achieve great muscle tone, cardiovascular conditioning, and fat loss in record time.

The Action Hero Diet Plan

As already discussed, your basal metabolic rate is the amount of calories your body would burn if it never moved. Of course, unless you're a coach potato in the true sense of the word, your body burns calories with everyday events such as walking and shopping and playing tennis. Therefore, your *total* caloric burn rate is determined by the sum of your basal metabolic rate plus all your daily activities. Your goal here is to train harder and build more muscle to burn more calories.

After determining what you currently eat and how many good calories you should consume, it's time to build a healthy menu plan. You must decide what you'll eat on a daily basis, and that requires planning ahead, which most people don't do. Consequently, temptations can easily sabotage weeks of hard effort. You're in charge, so don't accept any excuses for deviating from your food program. Think of it as setting an example for other people.

The Action Hero diet plans described here should help you get started. They're built around a 12-hour day.

BREAKFAST

I can't tell you how many times I've heard people say, "I can't eat so early in the morning." In today's rushed society, people often skip breakfast or grab a coffee and muffin on the go.

Here's a simple rule: Never leave the house without breakfast. After a night of fasting, your body needs food first thing in the morning for instant energy and to convert into building materials during the day ahead. *Plan for your meals in advance.* This may seem odd in the beginning, but you'll get used to the program. You probably know when all your appointments for the next day will be, right? Why can't you also plan your meals at the same time? It's not that difficult.

Make sure that breakfast is your biggest meal of the day; it should include 30 to 35 percent of your daily caloric intake. For your first meal of the day, you need macronutrients such as protein, carbohydrates, and essential fats. Choose food that's high in complex carbs or has a moderate amount of simple carbs and protein. Foods such as oatmeal, cereals low in sugar, egg whites, and fruit. Keep the fat content low.

If you work out in the morning, eat 2 hours beforehand or have a quick snack before doing your aerobic activity or weight-lifting regimen and then eat a *complete* breakfast after your workout. It could consist of a full-fledged meal replacement drink. Also—and this is important—*never wait longer than 2 hours after you wake up before eating.* That's why you eat that snack first thing before heading to the gym. The nutrients will nourish your body when it's craving them the most: after a night's sleep and before a kick-start workout.

If you don't work out in the morning—no cardio, no weights—then start your day with a complete breakfast. You might want to work out at lunchtime. (That's fine, but make sure you eat lunch after your workout.)

Sample Breakfast (700 calories)

A bowl of oatmeal, fruit, and fat-free milk

Five egg whites and one whole egg prepared with cooking spray

A small glass of pomegranate juice or piece of fruit

MIDMORNING SNACK

Depending on the total number of calories you're eating a day, your snack can range from an apple to a full-fledged meal replacement drink. If you worked out in the morning, then skip the midmorning snack. If you didn't work out but ate breakfast first thing, you can have a snack about 2 or 3 hours later.

Sample Midmorning Snack (300 calories)

A protein bar, protein shake, or piece of fruit, all depending on your total caloric intake per day

LUNCH

You should have this meal about 2 to 3 hours after your midmorning snack, or about 4 hours after breakfast if you didn't have a snack. The meal itself should be about the same size as your breakfast, that is, 30 to 35 percent of your total caloric intake. Because this meal falls relatively early in the day, your metabolic rate is still high enough to handle a large amount of calories.

Sample Lunch (600 calories)

A big sandwich with lots of turkey, lettuce, tomato, and mustard

Or a rice bowl with marinated chicken and a salad

Or a burrito with chicken, beans, rice, lettuce, and tomato

MIDAFTERNOON SNACK

Again, depending on the total amount of calories you're eating per day, this snack can vary from an apple or a handful of fat-free pretzels to a full-fledged meal replacement drink. In most cases, it will be a little higher in calories than your morning snack, because the interval between lunch and dinner is usually longer than the one between breakfast and lunch. This snack is also important, because it will curb your appetite later in the day, about the time most people begin craving chocolate or coffee. If you keep working at your job and don't give your body any nutrition, your mind and stomach will go crazy, and you'll be ready to scarf down a whole cow by the time 6:00 P.M. comes around. When people don't eat enough throughout the day, they invariably eat too much at dinner.

Also, this snack, in conjunction with lunch, is important if you plan to exercise after a long day of work. Even though you might not feel like working out then, it's probably the best time of day to do so, especially if your job involves a lot of desk work. Your mind might be tired, but you've been fueling your body all day with good food, and it's ready to

RESTAURANT STRATEGIES

During the first few weeks of your diet, you might find it easiest to avoid restaurants altogether. The good ones are designed to relax you, tempt you with rich food and lots of alcohol, and then politely lighten your wallet of a week's pay. The bad ones are designed to snag you when you're in a hurry and weak from hunger, gratify your desire for fat and sugar, and keep you coming back for more. Either way, they're not helpful when your body is adjusting to a sugar-free, low-fat nutrition plan.

However, once you've found your diet groove, there's no reason that you shouldn't enjoy a meal out once in a while. But, just as you do with your nutrition plan, you must have a strategy in place. Planning ahead works in restaurants, too.

First, do your homework. Find out what restaurants offer before you actually eat there. Drop by in the middle of the afternoon when things are quiet and ask to see a menu. Chat with the headwaiter and ask how they prepare the dishes that look good to you. Do butter and cream play starring roles in the dishes? Are the chefs food snobs who will scream and tear their hair out if you suggest a change to their works of art, or are they willing to work with you? Usually the better restaurants will prepare things to order—you just have to ask.

If you're in a situation where you don't have time to check out the menu before-hand—an important business lunch, say, or a spontaneous and promising date—then scan the menu for items you're already eating on your diet, and ask for those. (I don't think a restaurant exists that doesn't serve chicken.) Avoid elaborate meals smothered in sauces. Check out the appetizers for vegetable plates and order one in addition to your entrée. Go for lean meat without the added fat, or fish rather than fried foods, and ask that the salad dressing be served on the side and the butter left off your potato. Many of the vegetable dishes will be low-fat and creatively pre-pared, so pay attention to what's offered in that department.

If you're eating out at lunchtime, you have a little more leeway caloriewise, and you can do fine with a good-size gourmet sandwich (though make sure only lean meat goes in it and ask that they hold the mayo) or a bowl of rice, chicken, and vegetables. For dinner, you're best off with grilled lean fish and salad. Instead of wine, ask for bot-tled water like Perrier—the restaurant will probably be happy to supply it and charge you as if it were champagne. Otherwise, just go for your local purified tap water.

Don't be the least embarrassed about your nutrition plan when you're eating out. Just smile and say to the people at your table, "I've finally discovered what tastes good and makes me feel great." And be sure to thank the waiter and chef—they'll be more willing to accommodate you the next time you eat there.

explode. Make the effort. After a quick warmup, you'll feel your energy kicking in, and you'll be glad you decided to work out.

Sample Midafternoon Snack (200 calories)

A protein bar, shake, or piece of fruit

DINNER

This meal should be the smallest one of the day. The amount of calories given to protein should be the same as for the other meals, but the complex and simple carbohydrates count should drop virtually to zero, except for vegetables and salad. Your fat intake (which more than likely will come from the fat in the meat and the olive oil on your salad) should stay the same. Set aside about 25 percent of your daily caloric intake for dinner. Those of you who have higher metabolisms can include a moderate amount of complex carbs such as brown rice or a yam.

Always eat your dinner *after* your cardio workout or weight lifting. Not only will your body welcome the nutrition, but your metabolic rate will be elevated from an aerobic activity, and you'll burn the calories of the meal more efficiently. By reducing or even skipping the complex carbs altogether, you'll be burning extra calories from your stored fat reserves. Even better, because your metabolic rate will stay elevated for roughly 3 hours after your workout.

Sample Dinner (500 calories)

A large chicken breast or lean fish or a piece of lean red meat once a week, broiled, boiled, or steamed; small amount of rice; salad with olive oil and vinegar or steamed or lightly sautéed vegetables, or a combination of both

LATE-NIGHT SNACK

Eat a small amount of protein, and that's it. Just enough to stave off those hunger pangs through the night.

Sample Late-Night Snack (100 calories)

Soup (light chicken or vegetable made with fat-free or low-fat chicken broth)

Or a couple slices of turkey

Pick Your Plan

Here are three simple diet plans based on a man's height and his Action Hero weight goal. If you're a tall person, your height is important in determining how many calories you need to consume. You need more nutrition to support your body. Even though I promote designing your own diet, I supply you with these sample diets. Figure out which one is most appropriate for you.

THE 1,500-CALORIE DIET

This program is especially designed for men who are in the 5-foot-5 to 5-foot-7 height range and have an Action Hero weight goal of between 155 and 170 pounds.

Breakfast (500 calories)

Five egg whites, any style, and ¾ cup oatmeal with fat-free milk, Equal sweetener (or any other noncaloric sweetener), and one chopped-up banana or an apple

• Substitute for oatmeal: a cereal of equal caloric value, such as All-Bran, Grape-Nuts, Shredded Wheat, or Total

• Substitute for oatmeal *and* fruit: two slices of bread and a small glass of fresh pomegranate juice

Snack (150 calories)

10 to 15 almonds or cashews

Or one serving of fat-free pretzels

Lunch (400 calories)

A sandwich with whole wheat bread and turkey or chicken (you can add mustard, lettuce, tomato, and sprouts)

Or an all-white-meat chicken bowl and a small green salad

Or a small burrito with all-white-meat chicken, lettuce, tomatoes, and rice, but not at a fast-food chain—you should know better than that

Snack (180 calories)

A piece of fruit

Dinner (350 calories)

5 ounces chicken or turkey breast or 5 ounces fish (red snapper, cod, orange roughy, or halibut), and a baked yam or potato and assorted vegetables (mainly broccoli)

Snack (optional)

1 cup fat-free yogurt

Or two slices of turkey or chicken

THE 2,000-CALORIE DIET

This program is especially designed for men who are in the 5-foot-7 to 5-foot-9 height range and have an Action Hero weight goal of between 170 and 185 pounds.

Breakfast (605 calories)

Six egg whites (any style) and 1 cup oatmeal with fat-free milk, Equal sweetener (or any other noncaloric sweetener), and one chopped-up banana, an apple, or 10 raisins

• Substitute for oatmeal: a cereal of equal caloric value, such as All-Bran, Grape-Nuts, Shredded Wheat, or Total

ACTION!

Action Hero: Angelina Jolie

Career accomplishments: Angelina has appeared in a number of demanding action films but most notably *Tomb Raider* and *Tomb Raider 2.* She won an Academy Award for Best Supporting Actress in *Girl Interrupted.* Her long list of feature film accomplishments includes roles in *Beyond Borders, Life or Something Like It, Original Sin,* and *Gone in Sixty Seconds.*

Physical goals: Strong-looking body, with cut arms and shoulders in combination with good cardiovascular conditioning to endure the gruesome work schedule for the movie *Gone in Sixty Seconds.*

Training program: Just like for the guys, the basics of the Action Hero training system, with supersets and intervals on the bike, hard abdominal workouts, and aerobic activity to drop some more body fat from an already fairly lean body.

Results: I wish I'd had more time with Angelina to help her reach her full potential. Nevertheless, she reached her objectives to make her a prime candidate for the movie part. Watch her! She's badass!

Angelina and I had a great relationship in the gym, and she did unbelievably well with the workouts. She's strong, well-coordinated, driven, and responsive. These qualities represent all the elements necessary to build an Action Hero physique.

We worked out nearly every day and focused on different parts of her body. She did very few, mostly straight sets such as back followed by biceps, chest followed by triceps, legs by themselves, and shoulders followed by a light superset for arms.

Almost every workout she'd do the bike or slow-moving treadmill to stimulate the body to use what little fat reserves she had in order to get that crisp, cut, athletic look. Because of her hectic shooting schedule, we couldn't fit in as many workouts as I wanted, but Angelina made great progress.

For slender, athletic women, straight-set or high-intensity workouts can greatly improve muscle tone.

Snack (150 calories)

10 to 15 almonds or cashews

Or one serving of fat-free pretzels

Or a small granola bar

Lunch (600 calories)

A sandwich with whole wheat bread and turkey or chicken (you can add
   mustard, lettuce, tomato, sprouts, and one slice of provolone cheese) and
   a piece of fruit

Or a large all-white-meat chicken and rice bowl and a small green salad

Or a burrito with all-white-meat chicken, lettuce, tomatoes, and rice

Snack (150 to 200 calories)

A banana or a small granola bar

Dinner (500 calories)

6 ounces chicken or turkey breast or 6 ounces fish (red snapper, cod,
   orange roughy, halibut) and a baked yam or potato or small bowl of
   steamed rice and assorted vegetables (mainly broccoli)

Snack (optional)

1 cup fat-free yogurt

Or two slices of turkey or chicken

THE 2,500-CALORIE DIET

This program is especially designed for men who are in the 5-foot-9 to
6-foot-3 height range and have an Action Hero weight goal of between
185 and 200 pounds.

Breakfast (625 calories)

Five egg whites and one whole egg, 1¼ cups oatmeal with fat-free milk, Equal
sweetener (or any other noncaloric sweetener), and one chopped-up banana,
an apple, or 20 raisins

• Substitute for oatmeal: a cereal of equal caloric value, such as All-Bran,
Grape-Nuts, Shredded Wheat, or Total

Or a Jørgy shake (see page 68 for recipe). This one you should prepare the
night before, especially when you face a busy, early morning with no time
to prepare a normal breakfast.

Snack (300 calories)

20 almonds or cashews

Or two servings of fat-free pretzels, or a granola bar

Lunch (600 calories)

A sandwich with whole wheat bread and turkey or chicken—you can add
mustard, lettuce, tomato, sprouts, and one slice of provolone cheese

Or a large all-white-meat chicken and rice bowl and a small green salad

Or a large burrito with all-white-meat chicken, lettuce, tomatoes, and rice

Snack (250 calories)

One scoop of meal replacement supplement (Montiff) mixed in water

Or two bananas

Or a granola or protein bar

Dinner (600 calories)

7 ounces chicken or turkey breast or 7 ounces fish (red snapper, cod,
orange roughy, halibut) and a large baked yam or potato

And a bowl of steamed rice and assorted vegetables (mainly broccoli), a
salad with vinegar and olive oil, or a combination of both

Snack (100 calories)

1 cup fat-free yogurt

Or four slices of turkey or chicken

SAMPLE RECIPES

Instant Oatmeal with Blueberries and Star Anise

⅔	cup fat-free milk or water
1	1¼-inch piece ginger, peeled
1	star anise, whole
¼	cup instant oatmeal
¼	cup fresh blueberries

In a small saucepan, heat the milk or water with the ginger and the star anise. Add the oatmeal and stir. After the mixture cooks for about 1 minute, add the blueberries and cook for an additional minute. Done!

Scrambled Egg Whites with Cherry Tomato–Asparagus Salsa

½	cup cherry tomatoes, halved
4	spears asparagus, cut into 1-inch pieces
5	large basil leaves, coarsely chopped
1	teaspoon extra-virgin olive oil
	Balsamic vinegar
	Salt
	Black pepper
4	large egg whites

For the salsa, wash and cut the cherry tomatoes and place in a small bowl. In a small saucepan, bring 1 cup of water to a boil, add the asparagus, and cook for 1 minute. Drain and cool in ice water. Remove the asparagus from the water and add it to the cherry tomatoes. Add the basil and oil. Add vinegar, salt, and pepper to taste.

Scramble the egg whites until set in a large, nonstick skillet coated with cooking spray. Top with the salsa or add it to the skillet a minute or so before the egg whites are set.

Egg White and Fresh Dill Pita with Smoked Salmon and Asparagus

2	ounces smoked salmon, cut in thin strips
2	spears asparagus, steamed and cut into ¼-inch pieces
1	tablespoon fresh dill, chopped
4	egg whites, lightly beaten
	Salt
	Black pepper
1	pita, halved crosswise

Combine the salmon, asparagus, and dill and add to the egg whites. Add salt and pepper to taste. Heat a large nonstick skillet on high heat for about 30 seconds. Remove the skillet from the burner and spray with cooking spray.

Return the skillet to the burner and add the egg white mixture. Cook for 1 or 2 minutes until the egg whites are set. Heat the pita halves in a toaster for 30 seconds or until warm to the touch. Stuff the egg mixture into the pita halves and serve.

Jørgy's Famous Protein Shake

16	ounces water
1	cup fat-free Yoplait yogurt
1–2	cups instant oatmeal, uncooked
1	teaspoon olive oil
2–3	scoops Montiff meal replacement shake powder

Blend all the ingredients, let the mixture sit overnight in the refrigerator, and drink up.

This shake will deliver up to three meals, depending upon your total caloric intake. It will be perfect when you're stuck at the office or caught in traffic. Make sure it is in a container that will keep it cool.

The Urge to Splurge

It might help you to think of the Action Hero diet plan as a ballpark: It has room to move around in but also very strict boundaries. You can move within those boundaries, but under no circumstances can you step outside them.

I've been living on this diet for 23 years—no joke. Fortunately, I have a naturally high metabolism. However, by following this diet and using a little discipline, *any*body, whatever his or her metabolism, will see amazing results.

About the discipline: Don't get me wrong. I'm not a drill sergeant about this. You can and should give yourself a treat every once in a while, preferably on weekends. On the other hand, sometimes you'll feel so good about your personalized Action Hero regimen that you won't even have the urge to splurge.

However, some people like to eat those additional calories on weekends so their bodies and minds don't feel deprived. During the week, when you're dieting, your body has a tendency to slow down to adjust to the lower caloric intake. A weekend "splurge" boosts your metabolism so that when you start your diet again on Monday, your body continues to burn the calories, including those you had on the weekend, at the higher metabolic rate.

Sounds weird, I know. But it works.

When your body is running on all eight cylinders as a result of your AH program, it becomes an efficient fat-burning machine. During the week, when you eat only exactly what you need—maybe even less when you try to shed a few pounds of fat—your body adjusts to the reduced calorie count as a protective measure. Then on Saturday, your cheat day, your highly efficient mind/body goes into overdrive and starts to burn up all those extra calories.

Once Monday rolls around and you drop your caloric intake to AH levels, the body stays on the high level of calorie-burning capacity for a day or two. This creates a state of extra body-fat burning. By the time

Wednesday comes around, your body has adjusted and lowered its caloric burning rate to the level it was used to, the original caloric intake that you created when you designed your AH plan.

Come Saturday and Sunday, when you add an extra 100 percent of your dietary caloric intake (if you've been doing your AH plan and your body is in high gear), your body thinks, "Wow, I've got an energy supply to last forever." It'll then go into overdrive and utilize every single calorie that's being put into your system.

One note of caution: If you're too disciplined and stay on a low-calorie diet even through the weekends, your body will be so efficient that it will reduce its caloric burning rate, which will cause more harm than good. With this scenario, in order to lose more fat, you'd have to eat less and less the longer you were on the diet.

Fit Forever: My Weekly Action Hero Lifestyle

For most of my life, I've focused on eating right—the right foods and supplements eaten at the right times—and as I've told countless clients to do, I've stuck to it religiously. My diet—no, make that my lifestyle—sounds boring when you read it, but its effects over the long term have been nothing short of phenomenal.

I'm not going to argue with the results, and I never want to compromise the dramatic physical and mental well-being that I enjoy every day. Even at 38, I've never felt stronger, healthier, or more alert. I've never looked better—and that's according to the ladies and some of the guys who feel secure enough to compliment a fellow gym participant. I can tell you that this regimen truly has become a blueprint for my life.

Everything I've learned about good nutrition and that I tell my clients, I practice myself. And I mean *everything*, including being tempted to cheat on my diet every now and again. Okay, I admit it: I am and I do. But I'll get right back on the wagon and be good for a couple of months before I fall off again. Don't get me wrong: I still "cheat" on the weekends, as you'll see from the following schedule, but that's a legitimate part of the Action Hero lifestyle, as I've explained already.

Here's my typical weekly schedule. Not every day is the same, so I try to plan ahead. Being prepared really works in your favor as you follow the AH plan. You're far less likely to stray or slip up if you set yourself up to succeed and make sure you have the right food on hand.

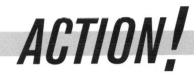

Action Hero: Cliff Shiepe

Physical goals: He wanted improved health and weight loss. I added in strength and athleticism.

Training program: Seven to 14 aerobic-activity sessions and on three occasions a reintroduction to weight lifting in its most basic and effective form.

Results: Cliff is proof that anyone can be an Action Hero if he or she tries. Besides losing the weight, Cliff became strong, healthy, and less stressed.

He had started by training with different trainers, but never really got the results he was after. He had eight different trainers before he read about the Action Hero training system in *Men's Health* and decided to give it a try.

When we started working out, he told me that one of his trainers had considered his goals "far-fetched" and said he'd never get lean; he didn't have the genetic disposition to become muscular and athletic.

After a lot of treadmill work, in particular pushing The Cart, and some heavy-duty Action Hero workouts, Cliff had lost roughly 35 pounds, doubled his strength, and was fast closing in on his target Action Hero goal weight. He also went up against all the odds and proved his ex-trainers wrong.

This is a guy, just like you, who probably had every excuse to fail in pursuing and obtaining his goal. Instead, he went for it and changed his life. He's everything he wanted to be and truly deserves the status of Action Hero.

Short, intense AH workouts are far better for muscle gain than long, less-intense workouts. Long, less-intense aerobic activity sessions are far better for fat loss than short, intense cardiovascular activity sessions. For more information on Cliff's experience, see page 234.

MONDAY, WEDNESDAY, AND FRIDAY (WORKDAYS)

6:00 A.M.—Upon awakening, I take 10 Montiff arginine (amino acid) capsules and a large glass of water.

6:30 to 7:30 A.M.—Train my first client.

7:30 A.M.—Five-minute breakfast break. I drink half of a Jørgy-style Montiff shake (recipe on page 68) during my first break (600 calories). I also take these other Montiff supplements: one Vitaminz, one Super C, and one B-Complete.

7:30 to 8:30 A.M.—Train my second client.

8:30 to 9:00 A.M.—Return home to pick up my daughter, Emma, and drop her off at preschool.

9:00 A.M.—Second 5-minute breakfast break. I drink the other half of my Jørgy-style Montiff shake (600 calories).

9:00 A.M. to noon—Train clients, sometimes as many as five during this 3-hour interval. When that happens, I train two simultaneously.

Noon to 1:30 P.M.—Pick up Emma (my little firecracker, my princess, my treasure) from preschool, play in the park, return home to make her and myself lunch and prepare a regular Montiff shake to take with me for the afternoon.

1:00 P.M.—Lunch. I have two potato buns with low-fat turkey patties and mustard. Occasionally, I'll add one slice of cheese (700 calories total). More Montiff supplements: one Vitaminz, one Super C, and one B-Complete.

1:30 to 6:00 or 7:00 P.M.—Another four or five clients. At 2:30, I run out to meet with my oldest client, Berton Steir, to train him at his office.

3:45 or so—On my way back to the gym, I reach into my cooler and have the regular Montiff shake I made earlier (300 calories).

6:00 or 7:00 P.M.—Arrive home, put the babies in the bath or shower, read them stories, and then it's nighty-night for them!

7:00 P.M.—Dinner. I usually have homemade teriyaki chicken with green vegetables and rice (500 calories). My wife, Angel, prepares this before I come home, so getting the meal on the table takes me about 5 minutes. Montiff supplements in the evening are the same as in the morning and afternoon: one Vitaminz, one Super C, and one B-Complete.

7:30 to 10:00 P.M.—For the last year and a half, I've been writing this book (what an experience!), so I'm busy with that until bedtime.

Note: Throughout the day I drink plenty of water, one Diet Coke, and one glass of pomegranate juice. Total calories for each day: 2,700.

TUESDAY AND THURSDAY

6:00 A.M.—As on other days, upon awakening I take 10 Montiff arginine capsules with a large glass of water.

6:30 A.M.—Breakfast. I eat 2 cups of oatmeal prepared with water, 15 raisins, a couple of squirts of light maple syrup, six egg whites, and one whole egg (800 calories). Supplements as usual.

7:00 A.M. to noon—Train five or six clients.

9:00 or 10:00 A.M.—I have a snack of a regular Montiff meal replacement shake (300 calories).

Noon—Lunch. I eat one of my "Jørgy Double Turkey Specials," which is a sandwich on whole wheat bread or baguette with turkey, lettuce, tomato, and mustard, and I drink a small glass of orange juice (500 calories). I get this from the sandwich/coffee shop across the street from my gym; the girls who work there know how I want it prepared. Supplements as usual.

12:30 to 2:30 P.M.—Train two clients.

2:30 to 4:00 P.M.—Pick up my son, Vincent, (who's the future of ice hockey) from school and play, most often ice hockey drills in the carport.

3:00 P.M.—Snack. If I planned ahead and prepared it, I have a Montiff regular meal replacement shake. Otherwise, I have the least harmful protein snack that the local grocery store sells. Usually that's a MetRx or Pure Protein bar, or an EAS meal replacement drink (about 300 calories).

4:00 to 7:00 P.M.—Train three clients.

7:00 P.M.—Dinner. I have turkey or chicken with rice and some kind of vegetable. Or I might get creative and make a huge egg-white omelet with leftovers in it, such as cut-up turkey patties, wild rice, low-fat cheese, spinach, and some pasta sauce (500 calories). I kid you not: It's delicious!

7:30 to 10:00 P.M.—Return phone calls, catch up on bookkeeping, or hang out with the wife and watch some TV.

Total calories for each day: 2,400.

I know, you noticed already: no workouts. Of course I work out—usually every other day, sometimes 2 days in a row. With my busy schedule, I don't have a set time for it, but I work out whenever I can. It seldom happens that I can't train 2 days in a row. Usually I gamble on someone canceling an appointment that day or being out of town. No matter what, though, even if I have to train at 7:00 or 8:00 P.M. after a grueling day working with clients, lifting weights, and so on, I'm always motivated to work out. Always. I think about what my lifestyle gives me in return for keeping it up day in, day out. I know that the hour I put in at the gym, tired or not, will make me feel and look like an Action Hero for the rest of my life. (By the way, I'll give you my personal workout plan later in this book.)

WEEKENDS

Just for the record, cheating on the weekends doesn't mean nonstop scarfing, munching, and eating until you can't move your body. Not at all! I eat what I like in moderate portions. But even with some of the high-calorie items I enjoy on Saturday or Sunday, my total caloric intake is never more than twice as much as what I'd consume on a weekday. In other words, I keep my indulgences under 5,000 calories a day. Here are my legal slipups.

Friday night: I'll have two small cheeseburgers with grilled onions and ketchup and a chocolate milkshake from In-N-Out Burger, a decent fast-food chain in California.

Saturday lunch: I'll make a large sandwich with fresh turkey, mozzarella, avocado, hard-boiled egg, lettuce, and mustard. I'll also have a carrot cake bar for dessert.

5

MEALS DESIGNED FOR AN ACTION HERO

HERE'S A LIST OF SAMPLE nutrition programs that I designed for my more famous clients and others, each of whom had specific goals in mind. This should give you an idea of what kinds of foods to put in your AH diet, although by now you should be able to design your own diet based on my suggestions.

When you follow a healthy meal plan, your body will burn fat and calories more efficiently. You'll also reap the benefits of having more strength, endurance, and energy every day.

Anthony LaPaglia—Ripped to Threads

This is the diet I recommended to actor Anthony LaPaglia, who headlines the procedural TV drama about the Missing Persons Squad of the FBI. At the time, he needed to get his fitness program up and running. By the end of 3 months, he'd lost weight and was a lot stronger.

BREAKFAST

A protein shake (whey protein, fat-free milk) and a banana

Or **five egg whites cooked with tomatoes and mushrooms, two pieces of toast, and a small glass of fresh orange juice**

Usually Anthony chose the solid food over the shake; he was on a break between projects, so he had the time to prepare his food in the morning.

MIDMORNING SNACK

Five fat-free pretzels (150 calories)

LUNCH

One broiled chicken breast with a large yam and some lightly sautéed assorted green vegetables

Or **steamed or broiled fish (such as orange roughy, halibut, red snapper, sometimes salmon) with one scoop of boiled brown rice, and salad**

Or **a sandwich with grilled chicken or turkey with lettuce, tomato, sprouts, and mustard**

MIDAFTERNOON SNACK (OPTIONAL)

1 cup fat-free yogurt

DINNER

A large green salad with chicken or tuna, bell peppers, cucumber, vinegar, and 1 teaspoon olive oil

LATE-NIGHT SNACK (OPTIONAL)

One piece of chicken or sliced turkey

Ben Affleck—Lean and Mean

This is the diet Ben Affleck applied to get ready for the movie *Pearl Harbor.* I can't say that Ben is ever in bad shape, because he's genetically so gifted, but he needed to get in Action Hero shape, and we had only 6 weeks before the first shoot.

PLAN AHEAD

When you're hungry, it's essential that you detach your emotions from food. To do this, you must plan ahead.

• As you do with work appointments, go through your weekly calendar and plan ahead for when you'll be eating, according to the Action Hero plan.

• Do your grocery shopping for the whole week and buy only the food items that appear on your nutrition program. Make the list before you go shopping.

• Make room in your weekly schedule to work out at least three times a week, even if only for 30 minutes per session. It's better than nothing.

• If you're on a long plane ride or traveling by car, always bring a healthy snack or a cooler with a sandwich, fruit, and the like. Or, even better, bring a Jørgy shake.

• Avoid all situations that steer you toward the wrong kinds of food.

UPON AWAKENING

A cup of coffee and a Golden Delicious apple

BREAKFAST

Six egg whites with vegetables, two slices of toast, and a small orange
juice (This was before I discovered pomegranate juice, which I now
recommend as well.)

Or a Jørgy shake

LUNCH

Two broiled chicken breasts and a scoop of rice with a small green salad

Or a turkey sandwich with lettuce, tomato, and mustard

MIDAFTERNOON SNACK

A protein shake, any kind with a ratio of 40-30-30 (carbohydrates-protein-
fat)

He was rehearsing a lot, so he or I would get a ready-to-go shake at
the local grocery store.

DINNER

Steamed fish with a medium baked potato, steamed exotic vegetables, and
a salad

LATE-NIGHT SNACK (OPTIONAL)

1 cup fat-free plain yogurt

Ben Affleck—Buffed and Ripped

This was a diet I designed for Ben Affleck after he came back from a movie shoot and wanted to get back in tip-top condition. As you can see, this diet was much stricter than the previous plan, with fewer calories. We had to get him in shape quickly, but responsibly.

BREAKFAST

Five-egg-white omelet with mushrooms and tomatoes, three to four slices of toast, and a small glass of orange juice

Or a Jørgy shake

Ben loved the shakes and had those three or four times a week instead of the omelet meal.

MIDMORNING SNACK

Five to 10 fat-free rice cakes

LUNCH

One large piece of broiled chicken with rice (similar to a Teriyaki Bowl) and a salad with low-fat dressing

Or a medium piece of steak (filet mignon) with a small plate of pasta marinara and steamed vegetables

MIDAFTERNOON SNACK

A regular Montiff protein shake

DINNER

**Steamed or broiled fish (cod, red snapper, swordfish, halibut) with about a
cup of rice (prepared) and a large green salad with vinegar and 1 teaspoon
olive oil**

LATE-NIGHT SNACK

A regular Montiff protein shake

A Young Man—Weight Loss, Muscle Gain

I drew up this simple weight-loss program for a 20-year-old man who
needed help losing weight. He not only lost 50 pounds, but being strong
already, he grew even stronger and healthier, ultimately achieving his
dream physique.

BREAKFAST

**Six egg whites with vegetables and 4 ounces oatmeal made with fat-free
milk and a banana**

MIDMORNING SNACK

A Pure Protein Bar (from Worldwide Sports Nutrition)

LUNCH

One large chicken breast and 1 cup boiled rice with vegetables

He used salsa or teriyaki sauce as seasoning.

MIDAFTERNOON SNACK

A protein shake with water

Or a WSN Pure Protein Bar

DINNER

Steamed or broiled fish (cod, red snapper, swordfish, or halibut) with a medium baked yam and salad (He used vinegar and 1 teaspoon of olive or canola oil as a dressing.)

LATE-NIGHT SNACK

1 cup fat-free yogurt

Jeff—Clean Up Your Act

This plan worked for a guy who at the time was approaching 40 and was 15 pounds overweight.

BREAKFAST

Six egg whites with vegetables and 1 cup oatmeal with a medium banana

MIDMORNING SNACK

Two scoops of whey protein with fat-free milk

LUNCH

Two broiled chicken breasts with a scoop of rice and steamed vegetables

Usually he would eat at a local Japanese restaurant with his colleagues. The restaurant people prepared this meal according to his personal dietary needs. Nice, huh?

***Or* a turkey sandwich with lettuce, tomato, and mustard**

When there was no time to break at lunchtime, he had his assistant pick up a freshly made gourmet sandwich from the grocery store.

MIDAFTERNOON SNACK

Two scoops of whey protein with fat-free milk

DINNER

Lean fish (broiled or grilled) with a medium baked yam and salad (vinegar and 1 teaspoon oil for the dressing)

Nicholas Curren—Get Lean

Nicholas was a young, strong, athletic type, but in need of a healthful diet. He even ran the Los Angeles Marathon twice. He wanted to get stronger and more cut. Here's the diet I designed for him.

BREAKFAST

Five-egg-white omelet with mushrooms, tomatoes, and onions, two pieces of sourdough bread (or substitute a bowl of oatmeal), and one apple

Nick made his breakfast every day, because he discovered it was a good way to start the day.

MIDMORNING SNACK

Low-fat pretzels

Or **one piece of fruit**

LUNCH

Here are a few choices I gave him while he was on the road.

A rice bowl with all-white-meat chicken and beans

Or **a burrito with double chicken, rice, lettuce, and salsa**

Or **a turkey sandwich with lettuce, tomato, mustard (no mayonnaise, no avocado, no cheese)**

MIDAFTERNOON SNACK

A small granola bar (not to exceed 200 calories)

DINNER

8 ounces of fish (grilled, broiled, steamed, or boiled), a baked yam, and salad or vegetables

LATE-NIGHT SNACK (OPTIONAL)

A couple slices of turkey breast wrapped around a pickle

N. K.—Ripped, Chiseled, and Rock-Hard

This nutrition program was designed for a successful businessman in his forties who liked to train almost too hard. His main objective was rock-hard abs (he had the abs—I felt them—but they were hidden underneath the fat).

20 MINUTES BEFORE BREAKFAST

Three Montiff Super-Sports amino supplements (Super-Sports is a blend of essential and nonessential amino acids that help rebuild muscle tissue after strenuous workouts and helps to maintain a positive nitrogen balance throughout the day.)

BREAKFAST

Six-egg-white omelet with vegetables (use cooking spray to grease the skillet), an English muffin with jam (his personal favorite), and a small glass of orange juice

MIDMORNING SNACK

One piece of fruit (choose one: apple, orange, tangerine, grapefruit, plum, yellow peach, mango)

These particular fruits are low on the glycemic index.

20 MINUTES BEFORE LUNCH

Three Super-Sports amino supplements

LUNCH

6 ounces turkey in a sandwich with lettuce, tomato, sprouts, and mustard

Or one large skinless chicken breast with one scoop of rice and steamed vegetables

Or a large salad with fresh tuna and two pieces of bread

MIDAFTERNOON SNACK

One piece of fruit (apple, orange, tangerine, grapefruit, plum, yellow peach, mango)

20 MINUTES BEFORE DINNER

Three Super-Sports amino supplements

DINNER

8 ounces fish (halibut, red snapper, sea bass, sole, tuna, or whitefish) with a small baked yam and steamed vegetables

LATE-NIGHT SNACK

1 cup fat-free yogurt

6

SUPER SPORTS SUPPLEMENTS

AS I BECAME MORE knowledgeable about the effects on the human body of weight lifting, nutrition, and even rest, I started wondering how I could use this information to improve my Action Hero training system. Supplements and steroids were an obvious consideration, but I didn't know much about either of them.

I lived in Holland at the time, and the owner of the gym where I worked had begun selling his own line of supplements. I didn't give it much thought at first, mainly because supplements had never affected my brother's physique one way or another—and not counting myself, he was the person I was coaching. Still, I was curious to learn more. I wondered if there were other supplements that could give *me* something . . . extra.

Thus began my research.

First I studied the individual components of supplements to see how they might assist me in preparing for my first national bodybuilding competition. I experimented with amino acids, multivitamins, and minerals. I only used products that actually "supplemented" my nutrition program, and I hold to that principle today. For instance, if I needed an extra boost of vitamins because of my restricted-calorie diet and pre-contest workouts, I'd use supplements.

This same concept applied to my intake of amino acids. If I suspected I wasn't getting enough protein in my diet, I'd take pure, pharmaceutical-grade, L-crystalline amino acids. Most amino acids come in both D- and L-forms, the letters standing for the direction in which the molecule's chemical structure spirals. Proteins in animal and plant tissue are made from the L-forms, so these supplements are most compatible with human biochemistry. (Remember, our bodies convert protein that we eat into amino acids to use for muscle building as well as brain and organ functions.)

A lot of people take supplements to support their inadequate nutrition program or replace good, wholesome meals, but this is completely the wrong approach. A supplement can't make up for an unhealthy diet. In my case, I decided to use the highest-quality food supplements I could find. They worked—as a *supplement* to my already sound diet.

Supplements That Sell Themselves

After experiencing the benefits of supplements firsthand, I moved to England to develop with two businessmen and a biochemist a line of supplements for recreational and serious athletes. Our business was called Peak Fitness for Sport, and we kept it simple: a line of multivitamins and minerals, B complex, vitamins C and E, and several amino acid combinations.

Most businesses try to convince people to buy their products, hard-selling them as the best of their kind on the market. I never did that. I believed in this line of supplements, so I packed up samples in my car and drove around the country, visiting hundreds of gyms.

Of course, owners usually were willing to listen to me, because my brother was one of the best and most popular bodybuilders in the world at the time. And I was his fitness coach. My attitude was literally, "Hey, if you don't trust me and you don't want to buy my products, then that's your loss." I also conducted seminars about nutrition and the proper use of supplements. I even supplied everyone with a well-balanced nutrition plan.

I wasn't surprised when people began buying the products, and I felt justified in my approach when they said the results from using them were amazing.

Most people assumed that the high-quality supplements I peddled were working "miracles" and were responsible for improving their health and energy by 75 percent or more. Of course, it wasn't the supplements that improved their health but rather the strength-conditioning and cardio workouts, along with a sound nutrition program.

Don't miss my point here: Supplements can help you gain that extra edge, but they'll never replace hard work, discipline, and perseverance, or a nutritionally sound diet.

You don't have to be a world-class athlete to take advantage of the benefits supplements provide. By adding vitamins, minerals, and even amino acids to your daily nutrition program, you'll gain more energy for your Action Hero workouts, not to mention a better quality of life.

I've taken supplements every day for the last 20 years. They've helped me maintain my health and physique, and I've convinced many of my clients to do the same. All have reported similar results. This

SEVEN REASONS FOR SUPPLEMENTS

1. Drinking hot coffee and tea or eating foods with hot spices can inflame the digestive lining, resulting in a drop in the amount of digestive fluids your body secretes and, consequently, a lowered ability to extract all the vitamins and minerals in the food you eat.

2. Alcohol very much hampers your body's ability to absorb vitamins and minerals. It also can severely damage your liver and your pancreas, both of which are vital to digestion and metabolism. And alcohol can damage the lining of your intestinal tract and adversely affect how your body absorbs nutrients. This can lead to sub-clinical malnutrition. Recommendation: B-complex supplement the night before a night on the town, because it can help counter the stress to your gastrointestinal tract.

3. As most of you know, smoking is one nasty habit that causes severe lung and cardiovascular damage. It also irritates the digestive tract. Recommendation: an extra 30 grams of vitamin C per cigarette. Vitamin C is one of the single most important vitamins for the immune system.

4. Many people get involved with fad diets (you might actually be on a fad diet as you read this book). Pick your poison. Most of them come and go, but they can have long-term negative effects, especially those diets that suggest you discard a particular food group, which can cause unnecessary strain to your body's immune system.

5. Cooking meat degrades protein and cooking vegetables oxidizes and destroys the vitamins that are vulnerable to heat. Other foods are so processed that the vitamins and minerals are completely gone. Recommendation: vitamins B, C, and E.

6. In many cases, when somebody has food allergies, whole food groups are removed from that person's diet. For example, many people are allergic to gluten or lactose, which once removed could cause low levels of thiamin (B_1), riboflavin (B_2), and calcium. Recommendation: calcium and magnesium in a 2:1 ratio and a B-complex supplement.

7. Stress can significantly up the need for vitamins, especially the Bs and Cs. Although it has a positive effect on your body, even an Action Hero workout routine exposes your body to stress. Think of what a tense couple of hours in gridlock traffic while you try to catch a plane might do.

doesn't mean you must become a fanatic pill-popper to succeed on the Action Hero program, however. Even a simple multivitamin supplement in conjunction with a healthy, nutritious diet will make a huge difference in the way you feel and the results you'll be able to sustain.

I always recommend supplements to my aspiring Action Heroes, as long as they have a clean bill of health or permission from a qualified doctor. Here's an overview of the most important ones to add to your daily routine. Remember, all the capsule amounts are based on my own recommendations to my clients.

Protein Shakes or Meal Replacement Supplements

These days, you can take your pick from a large variety of protein shakes and meal replacement supplements on the market. Some contain fat burners, protein absorbers, vitamins, creatine, and combinations of different types of protein. With so many supplements to choose from, it's daunting and time-consuming for most people to compare the subtle differences between these products.

With the Action Hero nutrition plan, all you have to find is a product that says "protein shake" or "meal replacement." No more, no less. Look for products that are based on whey and egg-white protein, and those where one serving delivers anywhere between 20 and 40 grams of protein. Given the recommended guidelines in this book, supplementing your diet with 20 to 30 grams of protein is about right.

Many manufacturers also make decent meal replacement drinks. Usually the ratios are 40 percent carbohydrates (predominantly complex), 30 percent protein (usually whey), and 30 percent fat (usually mostly unsaturated fat). This ratio's okay if you're on a calorie-restricted diet. But if you're on a 3,000-calorie diet, a 40-30-30 ratio would mean you'd need roughly 200 grams of pure protein. That's insane!

I usually use one of the higher-quality meal replacement supplements (for a tasty example, Jørgy's Famous Protein Shake on page 68). Prepare it with the right amount of protein—that is, between 20 and 30 grams—and then add pure oatmeal. You can cook it or just put it into a glass of water and chug it down. It sounds nasty, I know, but it makes the perfect meal if you're on the go or rushed in the morning. Of course, you can get creative and add fruit or yogurt to the mix. Make sure, though, that you count every calorie you put in your shake in addition to the meal replacement mixture. They add up quickly.

Recommended dosage: No more than one or two protein or meal replacement shakes per day. Don't get lazy and have a shake instead of a nutritious meal. Remember, a supplement is something you add to your program. Don't use it as a substitute for healthy food.

Multivitamins and Minerals

Even with all the proper foods in your Action Hero nutrition plan, you still won't ingest enough vitamins and minerals to recover from the good stress that you put on your body during workouts. Most people think the Recommended Dietary Allowance they read on food labels should be enough. And for most people, maybe it is. But time and time again, I've proven to my clients and their doctors that good, pharmaceutical-grade food supplements are the perfect combination for people maintaining an Action Hero workout routine.

What does a multivitamin supplement do for you? In short, it helps regulate all your bodily functions. It also helps protect you from free-radical damage by providing important antioxidants.

Look for vitamins and minerals such as vitamin A and beta-carotene, which are important for healthy skin; the fat-soluble vitamins D, K, and E, which are important for healthy bones and teeth and a healthy nervous system; and vitamin E, which is a powerful antioxidant.

Antioxidants help combat those nasty free radicals, which attack healthy cells and cause oxidation damage, similar to the way oxygen rusts metal. They weaken the immune system, break down or alter DNA, hasten aging, and contribute to many debilitating diseases. Some of the afflictions caused or aggravated by free radicals include cancer, heart disease, high blood pressure, rheumatoid arthritis, and strokes.

Antioxidants will protect healthy cells from free radicals. Some antioxidants do this by disarming the extra electrons on the free-radical molecules, while others neutralize them, converting them to harmless chemicals.

In short, a few capsules a day of these supplements will ensure that

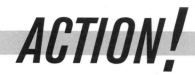

Action Hero: Billy Crudup

Career accomplishments: Billy began his career on stage in the Broadway production of Tom Stoppard's *Arcadia*. He was cast in the film *Sleepers* and appeared in Woody Allen's *Everyone Says I Love You*. His first big film role came with the indie movie *Inventing the Abbotts*. His first starring role was in *Without Limits*. Since then he's also starred in *Jesus' Son*, *Almost Famous*, and *Big Fish*.

Physical goals: To make him look and move like famed long-distance runner Steve Prefontaine for the movie *Without Limits,* which was produced by Tom Cruise.

Training program: As heavy a weight-lifting program as possible in conjunction with running, which he did with a running coach.

Results: Astonishing! Not a mission impossible! (See for yourself and watch the movie.)

When Billy walked into the gym, I knew I had my work cut out for me. At the time he was very thin and had never touched a dumbbell or barbell. My job was to make him look and feel like a world-class athlete in a record 6 weeks.

As he walked toward me, I noticed that he had all the potential in the world to

you have all the necessary vitamins you need to keep your body and mind functioning in harmony and free from the damaging effects of free radicals.

Recommended dosage: Take one capsule of the highest-quality brand multivitamin at breakfast, lunch, and dinner.

B COMPLEX

Personally, I've found B-complex supplements particularly helpful in regulating my digestion and keeping my skin clear. Thiamin (B_1) is necessary

build muscle, because even though he was thin, he had muscle tone everywhere and a very low body-fat percentage.

In order to look as much as possible like "Pre," Billy had to build up his chest, shoulders, and arms dramatically. We had to do this in the 6 weeks before he started his intense running schedule.

As Billy responded dramatically to the weight-lifting, diet, and supplementation program, he started building muscle quickly: In 6 weeks he gained 10 pounds without one additional ounce of fat added. He developed the chest, shoulders, and arms that Pre once had.

After the 6 weeks, he incorporated running with the lifting, and I readjusted his workout schedule to more of a maintenance program so he wouldn't lose all his hard-earned muscularity. The danger of overtraining is always apparent. Every third or fourth day, he took the entire day off. But some days he'd train with weights in the morning and run with his running coach in the afternoon. It was an intense schedule, but Billy came through like a pro.

One month later, he was off to Oregon to shoot the movie. Billy is one of my best students ever.

Heavy, straight-set bodybuilding workouts will give an already lean and slender person ultimate gain of muscle mass in record time.

for proper function of the nervous system and muscles, including the heart. It's involved in glucose metabolism and therefore essential for energy production. Riboflavin (B_2) and niacin (B_3) are important for energy metabolism, not only in the glycogen energy cycle but also for oxidizing fatty acids into energy. B_6 is important because it plays a critical role in metabolizing amino acids. It helps in the processes of building new muscle fiber. B_{12} is the granddaddy of them all. It helps your body form all cells, including red and white blood cells. Most of the other B vitamins are involved in maintaining healthy hair and skin and proper neurotransmitter health. They also help lower cholesterol and blood pressure.

Recommended dosage: Take one capsule of the highest-quality brand at breakfast, lunch, and dinner.

VITAMIN C

Vitamin C enhances the immune system. It's also a powerful antioxidant. We find vitamin C in fruits and vegetables. Mostly, though, it must be obtained through supplements. Cigarettes, alcohol, antidepressants, steroids, and stress in particular deplete our vitamin C reserves.

Vitamin C is a water-soluble antioxidant, so it can easily penetrate the inner parts of cells to provide antioxidant protection, whereas other antioxidants protect only cell membranes. Vitamin C also protects against nitrosamines, which are found in bacon and other processed foods. Not much to worry about here, though, as long as you're sticking to your Action Hero nutrition plan, right? Nitrosamines, by the way, are largely responsible for mouth, stomach, and colon cancers.

In short, with vitamin C you'll be less prone to illnesses. Not a bad thing to include in your daily menu.

Recommended dosage: Take one 1,000-milligram capsule at breakfast, lunch, and dinner. You can up the dosage to as much as 10,000 milligrams a day when you're sick with a cold. There's a lot of controversy about dosages, but if you have a clean bill of health and you don't have a weak liver, kidneys, or urinary tract, you shouldn't worry.

Amino Acids

Proteins, vitamins, minerals, carbohydrates, and fats are the essential nutrients that make up our bodies. They're responsible for growth and daily functions. When water and fats are eliminated, proteins make up 75 percent of the body solids that remain. They're essential components of muscle tissue, organs, enzymes, blood, antibodies, and neurotransmitters in the brain.

Proteins are made from amino acids, the "building blocks of life," and they regulate every biochemical reaction in the body. Every cell is comprised of proteins made from amino acids, and because cells are subject to deterioration, they must be replaced.

The most compatible amino acids for the human body are the L-forms. These are the ones that have muscle-building ability, and you'll want to add them to your nutrition plan as you work toward your ideal Action Hero physique. There are 20 amino acids, which the health and fitness industry categorize into essential and nonessential.

There are nine essential (L-form) amino acids your body requires and must obtain from food or supplements. It can't manufacture them from other amino acids. They are L-histidine, L-isoleucine, L-leucine, L-lysine, L-methionine, L-phenylalanine, L-threonine, L-tryptophan, and L-valine.

The nonessential amino acids are just as important but are categorized as nonessential because your body can make them from other amino acids. This biochemical conversion is called transamination. However, even though your body can make its own nonessential amino acids, it still needs the essential ones, along with other components such as vitamins, to do so.

The nonessential amino acids include L-alanine, L-arginine, L-asparagine, L-aspartic acid, L-carnitine, L-citrulline, L-cysteine, L-cystine, GABA, L-glutamic acid, L-glutamine, glycine, L-ornithine, L-proline, L-serine, taurine, and L-tyrosine.

Despite the fact that amino acids are found in all kinds of food sources—including whey, milk, and eggs—there's never a proper balance. By eating a well-balanced diet, we can try to equalize the supply and demand, but even then, given the high-intensity training and other aspects of a busy and stressful life, it's hard to maintain that balance over time.

Amino acid supplements are the ticket to establish a proper balance and ensure good health and longevity.

Which amino acids are the best? Pharmaceutical-grade, pure, crystalline amino acids comprise the singular L-form. It's a mouthful, but that's what you want to look for. Because these amino acids don't require digestion and are easily absorbed, your body can use them most effectively. Take them as capsules.

Crystalline L-form amino acids are derived from biological fermentation, extraction, and recrystallization for increased purity. This special fermentation process is similar to the way yogurt is made. The amino acids go through a filtration process until they're the purest, highest-quality crystalline amino acids, which are the most easily absorbed into the body.

AMINO ACID COMPLEX

Supplements with all the amino acids combined are usually powerful blends of the highest-quality crystalline L-form amino acids and other ingredients that help with uptake and transportation to cells. If you're serious about your health and workout regimen, then you'll definitely need to integrate an amino acid complex with your diet. It will help you get stronger, build more stamina and endurance, and allow your muscles to recuperate more quickly after an Action Hero workout.

During strenuous exercise, your body kicks into "amino acid catabolism" or amino acid breakdown. Supplementing before and after a workout provides an additional amino acid pool to optimize the anabolic (muscle-building) effects of exercise, which start to take place right after the workout and until the next workout.

Recommended dosage: Take three to five capsules of 700 to 1,000 milligrams each with a large glass of water or a small glass of pomegranate juice, depending on your total protein intake and body weight, 20 minutes before the three major meals and just before going to bed.

L-ARGININE

In my opinion, this is the best amino acid out there. Simply by taking it in a capsule form a couple of times a day in conjunction with my Action Hero nutrition program, I became healthier, stronger, and sexier in the true sense of the word. Trust me, it works.

Arginine is synthesized in the intestinal tract from citrulline, and its major food sources are nuts (peanuts, cashews, almonds, walnuts, and pecans). These are high in fat and aren't represented as a major ingredient in the Action Hero program. Arginine is the precursor for ornithine and is a vital part of the urea cycle, involved in the detoxification

JØRGEN'S SUPPLEMENT PROGRAM

AMINO ACIDS

Upon awakening: L-arginine

20 minutes before meals: Super Sport Amino

20 minutes before and after workout: L-leucine/L-isoleucine/L-valine

Before and after aerobic activity: L-carnitine

VITAMINS AND MINERALS

After breakfast: Vitaminz, B-Complete, Super C

After lunch: Vitaminz, B-Complete, Super C

After dinner: Vitaminz, B-Complete, Super C

OTHER SUPPLEMENTATION

Breakfast replacement: Jørgy shake (half of mixture)

Lunch replacement: Jørgy shake (half of mixture)

Snack: Montiff shake

Note: This is the most complete and effective supplement combination I've ever used. However, you can reap astonishing results just by using the vitamin and mineral combinations, combined with the Jørgy shake (whenever you don't have the time to prepare your Action Hero breakfast).

and elimination of ammonia. It's also important for protein synthesis, wound healing, and general immune system health. Eighty percent of seminal fluid is made of arginine. Recent studies suggest that it also plays a role in the reproductive system of women and increases their libido.

Recommended dosage: Take six capsules of 500 milligrams each upon awakening and 2 hours after lunch with a large glass of water or a small glass of pomegranate juice.

L-CARNITINE

This amino acid will help your body more efficiently mobilize fat to use it as an energy source—especially if you're on a calorie-restricted diet. Basically, it will help you lose the weight faster and more efficiently. L-carnitine is also a necessary component of heart and skeletal muscle tissue and essential for brain cells and healthy neurological function.

Recommended dosage: Take one or two capsules of 500 milligrams each before and after your aerobic session. If your aerobic session follows right after your high-intensity Action Hero workout, take one capsule before your workout and one after your aerobic session.

L-LEUCINE, L-ISOLEUCINE, AND L-VALINE (THE BRANCHED-CHAIN AMINOS)

This magical combo worked wonders for me during the preparation for my last bodybuilding competition. Not only did it give me more energy before and during my high-intensity workouts, but it also delivered the rebuilding blocks for my tired and torn-up muscles right after those workouts.

These amino acids don't have to travel from the stomach to the liver and kidneys before your body can use them. They move directly from the intestinal tract into the bloodstream, where they're delivered to muscles as an immediate energy source before strenuous activity or to rebuild muscle material afterward. In other words, instead of eating a full meal and waiting at least 2 hours for your system to digest it, you can have noncaloric building blocks delivered within 20 minutes of your workout. That's why these amino acids have such high anabolic and anticatabolic effects on muscles.

Recommended dosage: L-isoleucine: 1,000 milligrams; L-leucine: 1,000 milligrams; and L-valine: 500 milligrams before and after an intense AH workout.

CREATINE

I'm sure many of you have heard some bad news about this particular supplement. I've tried all the suggested dosages, and if you take creatine in the proper amounts, you shouldn't run into any of the so-called negative side effects. Instead, you can expect to have more strength and more stamina in your muscles during your high-intensity Action Hero workouts. However, I wouldn't recommend this product to anyone who isn't within 10 pounds of his or her ideal body weight, because creatine may give you that bloated feeling (of carrying around excess water weight). Don't get me wrong: It's a powerhouse supplement, but I believe people need to earn the right to use more supplements.

Creatine is a natural substance found in muscle tissue and made by your body with the help of enzymes, L-arginine, and other amino acids. The body can make about 2 grams of creatine on its own per day, and 95 percent of that is stored in muscle tissue. It's then synthesized in the liver. Also, you can find creatine in foods such as beef, salmon, and tuna, but only in very small quantities.

Recommended dosage: Take 1 to 2 grams with water, four times a day. You can always take more, spread evenly throughout the day, but never use more than what's suggested on the container. And always make sure that you use the highest-quality creatine monohydrate powder on the market.

THE ACTION HERO
WORKOUT

7

THE PHYSICAL LOAD

SADLY, MOST PEOPLE who buy expensive gym memberships start out with the best intentions but quickly falter and give up. Why? Because they haven't a clue how to work their bodies efficiently. They overdo it, strain or injure themselves, and grow discouraged. Without wanting to, they fall back into their old unhealthy routines and figure that an Action Hero physique just isn't possible for them.

However, with the proper training system, any body can become strong and healthy, and that includes yours. Not that your body will magically swell with muscles after only a few workouts. But internally you'll begin to notice signs: an overall sense of well-being and, in particular, muscular health; reduced stress and a sense of calm after each workout; and abundant energy when you wake in the morning that remains with you throughout the day. You'll actually begin to feel your body working and the blood rushing to and from your muscles after each workout.

Before you begin training, though, you must "find" your body. By that I mean you must discover firsthand how it functions, how it responds to different exercises, and what sort of workout cycle works best for you and your lifestyle.

Most people set themselves on the wrong path to a healthy body and lifestyle. They start out by training very hard and continue increasing their workouts until, inevitably, they hit the proverbial wall. Even though their intentions were good, they overtrain and cause themselves possibly countless physical and mental injuries.

To avoid this trap, you must know where to start, when to rest, how much exercise is too much, and a lot more. I've trained hundreds of clients with different genetic makeups, and I've designed countless safe, effective workouts for all of them. These routines won't get the better of you; they'll just make you better. And they're the ones you can follow for the rest of your life. I'll share them with you later in this chapter.

Warm Your Body for Energy

Always warm up on a bike, treadmill, or other cardiovascular machine for 5 to 10 minutes before you begin your AH workout. This will increase your circulation, which will boost your energy, and also get your adrenaline flowing. Mild stretching before a workout is also a good idea. Don't overdo it, though, because you'll relax your muscles, which is exactly what you *don't* want to do. It's all about contracting, not relaxing, the muscles. Stretching for more than 2 minutes after a warmup is a waste of time.

Follow your cardio warmup with weight-lifting warmups. Your first set should be performed at about 50 percent of your maximum capacity, which I define as whatever weight you can lift easily at least 12 times. The second warmup set should be at about 65 to 75 percent of your max, which I define as any weight that you can lift with a moderate amount of effort 12 times. If you're training at 85 to 95 percent of your capacity, execute two warmup sets like this before virtually every AH workout.

At this point you should be ready for your "cruise" sets (85 to 95 percent of your capacity), which I define as any weight you can barely lift 12 times with perfect form. As long as you can stay between 8 and 12 reps with maximum effort, you'll get stronger and more toned muscles.

Tips on Training

Make sure that form, that is, the execution of an exercise, is *never* compromised. If you need to drop the amount of weight you're lifting in order to execute an exercise in proper form and reach 8 to 12 reps per set, then so be it. Improper training causes harm to both joints and ligaments, and it creates a false sense of strength.

Before you embark on any weight-lifting routine, first find the best range of motion of each exercise. For example, when executing a barbell curl, always begin the exercise with your arms fully extended down the sides of your body. As you curl the weight, keep your upper arms close to your torso and perpendicular to the floor. At the peak of the movement, squeeze out the last "pump" of your biceps. Then lower the weight slowly and with control, resisting the gravitational pull of the weight, until the barbell finally touch your thighs. Don't sacrifice form. Ever. You control the weight; the weight should never control you.

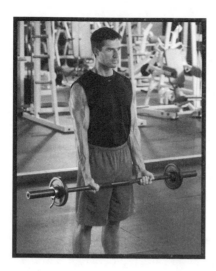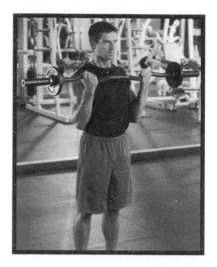

Let's say, for example, you're doing a high-intensity set (HIS), which I'll explain in more detail in this chapter. This is what the sensation should feel like: Rep 1 feels great. Rep 2 feels good. Rep 3 taxes your muscles. Rep 4, and you're finally awake. Rep 5, and you're struggling. Rep 6, and it's not getting any easier. Rep 7, and you're thinking to yourself, "I'm not quitting yet." Rep 8, and now you definitely feel the burn. Rep 9, and it's burn, baby, burn! Rep 10, and you've had just about enough. Rep 11, and you're too close to fail.

Your last repetition should be executed in exactly the same form as your first repetition, even though you'll feel more fatigued toward the end of the set. Any variation, and you'll defeat the purpose of the exercise. Rep 12 and yes! Success!

Start every first exercise of a new muscle group with a light weight, first executing the movement in proper form, before increasing resistance. It's no different than a long-distance runner who sets his pace in the beginning of the race and finishes with that last burst of energy. Believe me, he'll tell you that first and last mile may appear the same, but they certainly didn't feel the same. Yet he maintained the same running form throughout the entire race.

Same concept applies to your weight lifting: Always maintain the same, proper form throughout the entire set. Your physical strength may diminish near the end of the set, but your mental strength needs to stay strong. Use this to push yourself to do an extra rep, an extra set, or through the entire workout. A lot of highly driven people will do anything to get results fast, but often they do too much, too soon—which leads to burnout, undesirable results and, even worse, illness and injury. More isn't always better, especially when it comes to strength conditioning.

Once you've learned to execute all exercises in proper form, next find your body's frequency cap. Frequency refers to the number of workouts per cycle (a cycle refers to the time it takes for you to train all major muscle groups, according to a specific sequence). I don't believe you have to train your whole body once or even twice per week. Why? Because it takes longer for your legs, for example, to recover after a gruesome workout than your arms. If it takes 4 days for your legs to recover after an AH workout, why would you ever train your legs twice or even three times per week?

Lastly, each person has to figure out how much rest he needs between workouts. General rule of thumb: 4 days' rest for an intense leg workout, 3 days' rest for back and chest, 2 to 3 days' rest for shoulders, and roughly 48 hours for biceps and triceps. (Don't worry, I will give you all the cycles you'll ever need a little farther along in this chapter.)

I've listed all the exercises you'll ever need in this chapter, along with detailed descriptions of how to execute them in proper form. Understand that each additional rep executed in proper form will dramatically increase your chances of building an AH body.

Cruising Along

Your first set on cruise weight, or high-intensity set (HIS), should be relatively easy, although I really don't mean "easy" in the normal sense, because by reps 11 and 12, you should be tired. Your second set on cruise weight should be more difficult, because your fatigue level will start to kick in at this point.

Because your strength diminishes from set to set, the actual cruise weight feels heavier with each rep.

It's at this point that your mental strength must stay strong. Your goal is a second, or sometimes even third, set on cruise weight. Even if you feel you can't squeeze out another 12 reps, go for it. You have the physical strength that your mind allows. (*Note:* You might want to consider a spotter, or someone to help you, just in case you can't do that last bench or leg press.)

Heavy Lifting: Working the Percentages

In my workouts, I always talk about percentages instead of weight. This allows you to figure out your warmup set, your second warmup set, and the all-important cruise set.

50 PERCENT OF YOUR PHYSICAL CAPACITY (FIRST SET)

The first set of a heavy workout should always be a light one, what I call a 50-percent-warmup set. The percentage represents not only the amount of weight you're lifting, but also the number of reps you execute.

Take barbell curls, for example. For a light set, you'll want to select a weight that feels comfortable, one that doesn't require much strain during the first 5 reps. By the time you've performed 12 reps, you might feel a slight burn or nothing at all.

Warmup sets get the blood flowing to the muscles, joints, and ligaments. Your mind is also getting ready to perform. Use this set to practice your form: elbows close to the sides of your body; back muscles firm; abs, legs, and butt muscles clenched for stability.

People who consistently train at a low intensity typically spend 2 to 3 hours in the gym, four to five times per week. But high-intensity resistance training—otherwise known as weight lifting, bodybuilding, or body sculpting—is the key to an Action Hero physique. This sort of training creates muscle awareness in the body for the muscles specifically trained, but even more for those keeping your body stable and secure while you execute the move.

70 PERCENT OF YOUR PHYSICAL CAPACITY (SECOND SET)

The second set of a heavy workout should be done with a respectable amount of weight. I call this the 70-percent-warmup set. Use it to gauge how strong you feel that particular day. Your lifting capacity will vary, so don't expect to lift the same amount of weight you did during your previous workout, even for the identical exercise that works the same muscle group. Some days you'll just feel stronger than on others.

Once again, using barbell curls as the example, with this second set you definitely should feel a tightening of the biceps muscles right away. After roughly 7 reps, you'll feel a pump to the biceps as these muscles react to the weight.

Somewhere between reps 8 and 12 you should start to feel fatigued as your blood rushes to your biceps. At this point you'll know what your cruising weight on each exercise will be.

85 TO 95 PERCENT OF PEAK CAPACITY, OR CRUISE WEIGHT (THIRD SET)

The third, fourth, and sometimes fifth set of a heavy workout will determine the effectiveness of your routine. These are the 85-to-95-percent-of-your-capacity sets, or HISs, and the ones that will create the results you want.

Right after your first and second set, you're in the best shape to lift the most weight because you haven't reached a state of fatigue or muscle exhaustion. So for these sets, use the maximum amount of weight you can while maintaining proper form. Execute no fewer than 8 reps and no more than 12. If you can do only 7 reps with the weight you've decided upon, then you're close to exhaustion. Squeeze out one more rep, maybe even two, if you can. The set should leave you completely taxed.

Even if you're weaker than you thought, and you're disappointed that you couldn't lift the amount of weight you wanted to, your body nevertheless worked at 85 to 95 percent of its capacity—probably closer to 95 percent if you really pushed hard to reach rep 12. You're going to reap the benefits of that, regardless of the amount of weight you lifted. Take a break if you want, then do another set of 8 to 10 reps. Try for two or sometimes even three sets at 85 to 95 percent of your capacity.

Let's review.

50 percent of peak capacity (first set)	**12 reps**
65 to 75 percent of peak capacity (second set)	**12 reps**
85 to 95 percent of peak capacity (third set)	**8 to 12 reps**
85 to 95 percent of peak capacity (fourth set)	**8 to 12 reps**
85 to 95 percent of peak capacity (fifth set)	**8 to 12 reps**

Of course, these are only guidelines to get you started. If, for some reason, you're in the middle of a workout and doing more reps than you had planned, just remind yourself to stay in that all-important 85 to 95 percent of peak capacity range.

Body Sculpting:
Dividing and Defining Exercises

Before we get to the actual workout cycles and how to construct your own AH workout, allow me to explain the exercises that are needed to develop a defined, muscular, and athletic body. I've divided them into three categories: basic, concentration, and isolation. Each has its own place and function in your AH workout.

The basic exercises get you started, warm the muscle groups you're intending to train, and thereby avoid the risk of injury. Execute these exercises first, working as intensely as possible at 85 to 95 percent of your capacity while maintaining correct form. This should warm your muscles from all angles, and it will lay the foundation for a top-notch high-intensity workout, which will help you achieve that AH physique.

For example, let's say the Action Hero workout for a particular day focuses on your chest muscles. Instead of focusing on specific exercises for this area, such as Pec Decks, Butterfly Machine, or Cable-Cross Machine, aim for a presslike exercise such as the Flat Bench Dumbbell Press or the Incline Bench Dumbbell Press. That way you can warm up not only your pecs, but also other joints and muscles involved in the workout, such as your shoulders, elbows, and the muscles overlapping those joints, the front deltoids and triceps.

Later on in your workout you will do the concentration or isolation exercises. These don't take as much weight to reach total muscle exhaustion, especially now that you're done with the basic exercises. You've pre-exhausted the muscles to start the process of stimulating the muscle to growth and development. It is a matter of bringing the muscles to complete "failure" to induce maximum muscle growth. Keep reminding yourself: Your failure is your success.

After you have laid the groundwork for a rewarding workout with the basic exercises, move on to the concentration exercises to really work a particular muscle group. Machine exercises are the best way to concentrate on specific muscle groups. For one thing, you don't have to watch your balance, a concern as your muscles get closer to the point of complete exhaustion. The machines themselves aren't difficult to operate, whereas free weights need more coordination. Sets should be executed at 85 to 95 percent of peak capacity.

Isolation exercises work the specific muscle groups you want to train, with minimal help from secondary muscles. With these exercises, you really tax specific muscles. By using light weights, strict form, and about 15 reps, you'll get the pump of your life—if you perform the exercises at 85 to 95 percent of peak capacity. You have to keep pushing yourself until the end of the workout.

The Major Muscle Groups and Their Exercises

In the following section, you'll be introduced to all the exercises that will help you to construct your own AH workouts in accordance with your chosen workout cycle. I use these exercises in all my Action Hero workouts.

MAJOR MUSCLE GROUPS/EXERCISES

Chest

Flat/Incline Dumbbell Press	B
Flat/Incline Smith Machine Press	B
Vertical Bench Press Machine	B
Flat/Incline* Fly	C
Flat/Incline* Smith Machine Press	C
Pec Deck or Butterfly Machine	I
Cable-Cross Machine	I

*Choose a flat exercise if you started with an incline exercise, and vice versa.

Triceps

French Press	B
Overhead Dumbbell Extension	B
Triceps Pushdown	B
Overhead Rope Extension	C
Dippy	C

Back

Pulldown (medium or narrow reversed grip)	B
Low-Pulley Row	B
Lying T-Bar Machine (supported)	B
One-Arm Row (advanced)	B
Lat Pulldown (wide grip)	C
Chinup or Gravetron-Supported Chinup	C
Vertical Pull Machine	C
Cable-Cross Pulldown	I
Lat Flex	I

Biceps

E-Z Barbell Curl	B
Basic Straight Barbell Curl	B
Alternating Dumbbell Curl	B
Speedy Alternating Dumbbells	C/I
Straight Barbell Curl	C/I
Preacher Curl (advanced)	C/I
Cable Biceps Curl (advanced)	C/I

Shoulders

Shoulder Press Machine	B
Seated or Standing Dumbbell Press	B
Front Press on Smith Machine	B
Upright Dumbbell Row	C
Upright Row (straight bar/cable)	C
Seated Bent-Over Laterals with Dumbbells	C
Rear Deltoids with Cables	C
Rear Deltoids on Fly/Rear Deltoids Machine	C
Side Laterals (dumbbells or cables)	I
Front Laterals (dumbbells or cables)	I

Legs

Leg Press	B
Squat	B
Dumbbell Squat	B
Stiff-Legged Deadlift	B
Sissy Squat	C
Lying/Seated Leg Curl	C
One-Legged Skater Lunge (on bench)	C
Cross-Step Lunge	C
Lunge on Smith Machine	C
Leg Extension	I
Butt Squeeze	I

Basic (B)   Concentration (C)   Isolation (I)

Chest BASIC EXERCISES

Flat/Incline Dumbbell Press
Flat/Incline Smith Machine Press
Vertical Bench Press Machine

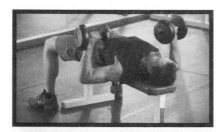

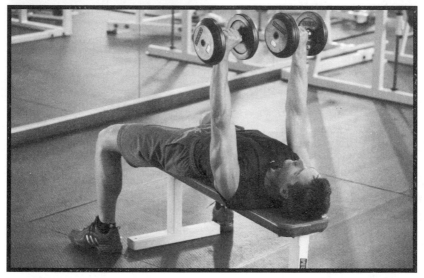

FLAT DUMBBELL PRESS

With both the Flat and the Incline Dumbbell Presses, make sure that your upper arms stay perpendicular to your upper torso and that, as you lower the weights, your elbows and upper arms stay under the dumbbells. Your upper back should be slightly arched, your butt and shoulders placed solidly on the bench, and your neck in a neutral position. Let your eyes, not your whole head, follow the weights. As the weights reach your chest, concentrate on keeping your chest contracted, and then drive the weights up. A good reminder is to push your elbows as close together as possible.

Tip: Always keep your feet placed solidly on the floor, slightly wider than the width of your shoulders. As you begin the exercise, put the pressure forward on your feet; this keeps you rock-solid in the right position.

INCLINE DUMBBELL PRESS

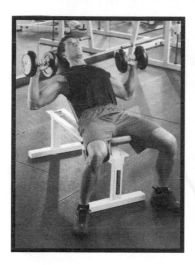 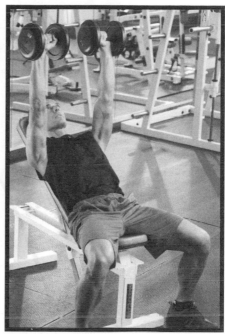

FLAT/INCLINE SMITH MACHINE PRESS

(NOT SHOWN)

This machine is designed to isolate the chest muscles without your having to worry much about balancing a heavy bar or a set of dumbbells. The positioning of your body on the bench is basically the same as when you do a dumbbell press. For the Flat Smith Machine Press, make sure that the bar touches your body on the lower part of your chest muscles. For the Incline Smith Machine Press, the bar should touch your body 2 inches below the top of your chest muscles.

VERTICAL BENCH PRESS MACHINE

(NOT SHOWN)

Make sure the grips are positioned at lower chest level—adjust the seat accordingly. Keep your shoulders tight and don't let them wander up toward your ears. It helps if you keep your latissimus dorsi muscles (in your back) tight. As far as your positioning and contracting the muscles targeted, it's the same principle as with the other presses.

Chest CONCENTRATION EXERCISES

Flat/Incline Fly
Flat/Incline Smith Machine Press

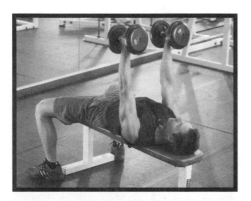

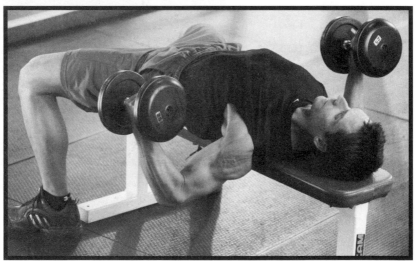

FLAT FLY

As a concentration exercise, the Flat or Incline Fly is probably the most effective chest exercise, if properly executed. Raise the dumbbells to arm's length over the chest, and fully extend your elbows. Make sure the palms of your hands are facing each other, and keep them roughly 6 to 8 inches apart. As you lower the weights, bend your elbows in conjunction with the descent of the dumbbells. Balance the dumbbells over your elbows so that your hands are above them. Don't go any farther than chest level. Control the weights, and push them back up for 1 complete rep.

INCLINE FLY

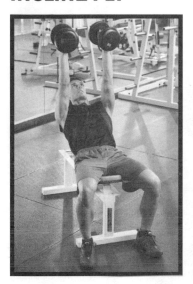
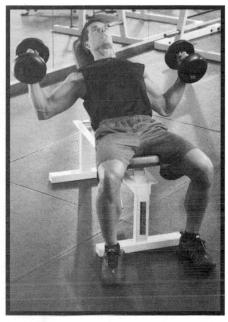

FLAT/INCLINE SMITH MACHINE PRESS

(NOT SHOWN)

This machine is designed to isolate the chest muscles without your having to worry much about balancing a heavy bar or a set of dumbbells. Personally, I like to perform a dumbbell exercise in the first part of my chest workout, followed by the Smith machine.

The positioning of your body on the bench is basically the same as when you do a dumbbell press. For the Flat Smith Machine Press, make sure that the bar touches your body on the lower part of your chest muscles. For the Incline Smith Machine Press, the bar should touch your body 2 inches below the top of your chest muscles. You could try a tighter fit by having the bar touch your chest just below the clavicle bone. It stretches out the muscle more and puts a greater strain on the muscles, but this variation is for Stage Three athletes only!

Chest ISOLATION EXERCISES

Pec Deck or Butterfly Machine
Cable-Cross Machine

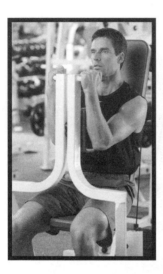

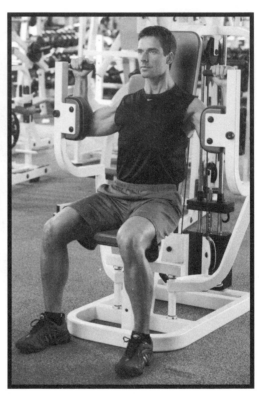

PEC DECK OR BUTTERFLY MACHINE

The Pec Deck somewhat simulates the dumbbell fly. Because you're using a machine, your body movement is minimal, and you're therefore putting all the stress of the resistance on the chest muscles. That's why I include this exercise in the isolation category. Never try to overdo it with this exercise. I always recommend at least 15 reps. Also, never attempt the machine's full range of motion; you'll put too much unnecessary strain on your already fatigued shoulder joint.

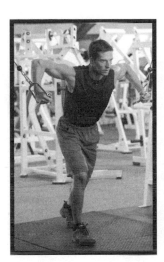

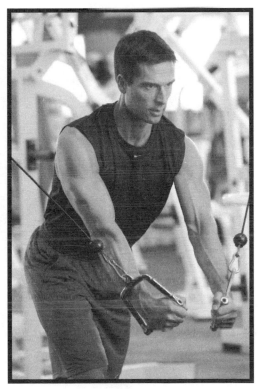

CABLE-CROSS MACHINE

Using the cable-cross machine is a great way to achieve maximum isolation of the lower and upper parts of the chest. By varying the position of your body and stance, you can create different angles, which stress the muscles in different ways. Make sure your elbows are bent when your hands are at the sides of your body and straight with about 3 inches between them when they're in front of you. As a variation, cross your forearms to the point where your elbows are almost extended and actually touching each other. This is called *peak contraction*.

Triceps BASIC EXERCISES

French Press
Overhead Dumbbell Extension
Triceps Pushdown

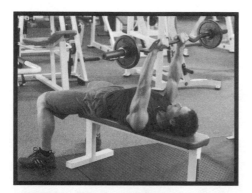

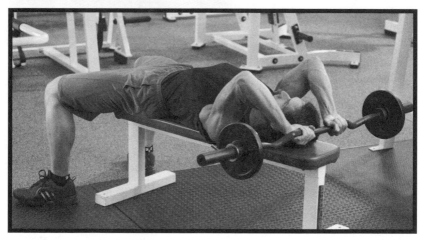

FRENCH PRESS

This is the most complete triceps builder because you're using all three heads of the triceps: long, short, and medial. Use an E-Z bar, if you can. At first, bring the bar in front of your chest with straight arms, bend your elbows, and lower the weight past your head. Try to keep the upper arms perpendicular to your body, except when you pass your head. When you touch the bench behind your head, move the weight all the way up again, only this time in front of your nose. Complete the set.

Tip: If you don't have a training partner, you can always leave a little space open on the bench behind your head where you can leave the bar at the end of the set.

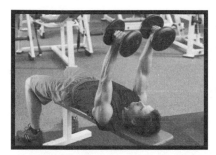 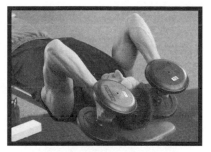

OVERHEAD DUMBBELL EXTENSION

Instead of an E-Z bar, use dumbbells to do the previous exercise. This can be an excellent exercise, because you have a little more mobility; you can actually move your hands around for better comfort, especially if the bar hurts your wrists.

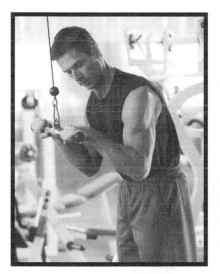 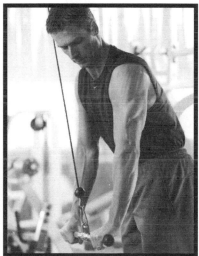

TRICEPS PUSHDOWN

With the pushdown exercises, you can use all kinds of bars. I prefer the straight bar, with either a medium or narrow grip. As you start the exercise, make sure your elbows are close to your torso and that your upper arms are perpendicular to the floor. Lean slightly forward, so that your upper body is in front of your hips, giving you adequate space to push the bar down and extend your elbows, without any obstruction from your legs. It helps to extend your legs by flexing your quads, butt muscles, and abs to avoid any hyperextension of the spine. As you let the weight go up again, don't lose control, but resist until the bar reaches your chest. Then push down again.

Triceps CONCENTRATION EXERCISES

Overhead Rope Extension
Dippy

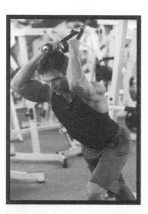

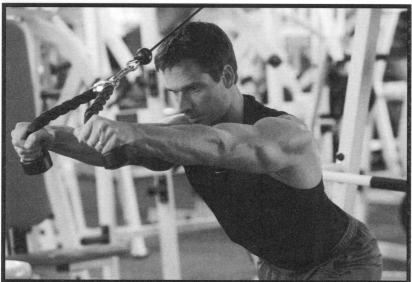

OVERHEAD ROPE EXTENSION

As with the pushdowns, with this exercise you'll "push" the weight out. But because you're using an overhead rope, you can place much greater stress on the other part of the triceps by bending the rope to the full extension of your arms. By the time you do 10 reps of this particular exercise, your triceps will be on fire. It's at this point that you should push for another 5 reps, if you can.

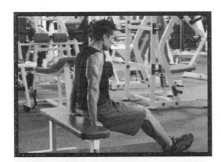

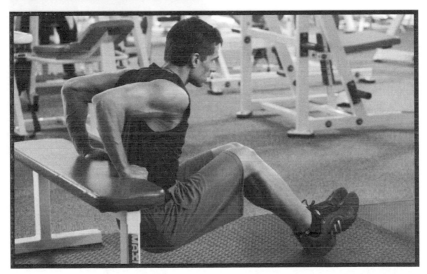

DIPPY

Put both hands on the edge of a bench, supporting your body weight. Face away from the bench, with your legs out in front of you. Move your body up and down by bending and straightening your elbows. Make sure you keep your back close to the bench and that you don't start wandering; it'll put too much unnecessary strain on your shoulder joint.

As a variation, place your feet on another bench. Only do this variation if the first Dippies don't deliver enough tension on the triceps by the end of the set. You can even go so far as to have your training partner or fellow gym member place a plate on your lap for additional resistance.

Back BASIC EXERCISES

Pulldown (medium or narrow reversed grip)
Low-Pulley Row
Lying T-Bar Machine (supported)
One-Arm Row (advanced)

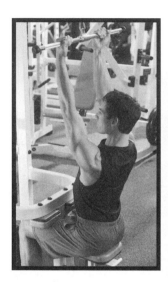
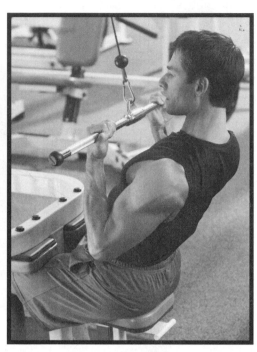

PULLDOWN (MEDIUM OR NARROW REVERSED GRIP)

For safety reasons, I prefer to do *all* pulldown movements to the front of the body. It's a two-way movement: You start with arms completely extended, then you move your body as you start the exercise to a 45- to 60-degree angle. Follow this with a pull using the backs of your arms, locking up the body as you're pulling the weight down to the chest. As you reach the chest and go back up again, move the body forward to a neutral position. Make sure that each part of the movement smoothly follows the other for an even flow. Repeat.

It's a great exercise to do intensely as a first exercise, because it warms up not only your lats (the prime movers) but also your biceps, lower traps, and rhomboids.

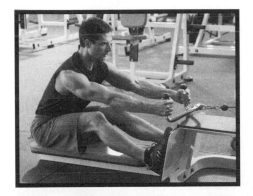

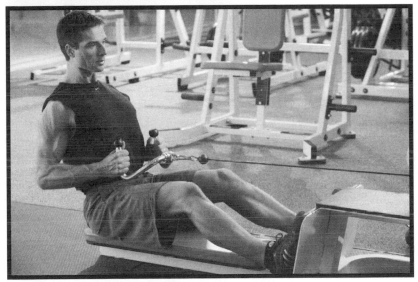

LOW-PULLEY ROW

This is one of my favorite exercises, because it works all areas of the back—including lats, lower and midsection of the traps, rhomboids, and lower back. If you perform it correctly, you can use a lot of weight and make your back as strong as a steel beam. When you have the bar in your hands, usually in a fish-bone grip, make sure that you always have a slight arch in your lower back and your knees are slightly bent. As you start moving the weight, move it at first with your upper body moving backward. As you reach the "one o'clock lock" (see bottom photo), start pulling with your arms and aim the bar just underneath your rib cage. Keep arching your lower as well as your upper back and contracting your lats, those big wings on each side of your body that give you that desirable V-shape.

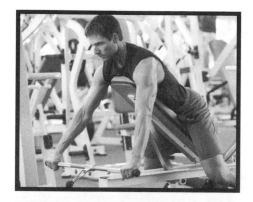

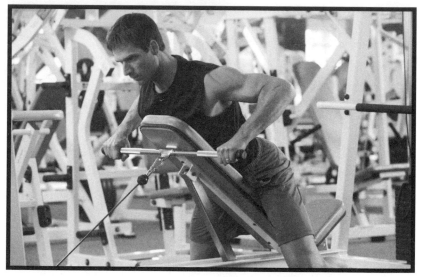

LYING T-BAR MACHINE (SUPPORTED)

This is also one of my favorite exercises, not only because it's a safe exercise but also because it's a great strength and muscle builder. Position yourself on the bench with your head and neck past the chest support, and use one of your favorite wide grips. Put your feet on each side of the machine—*not* on the platform that came with the machine. When you put your feet next to the machine, you're better able to arch your back and put more stress on the actual muscles that you're training.

Extend your arms, but don't fully stretch out your upper body. Keep the shoulder area tight and your upper and lower back arched. Pull the weight toward your chest and keep arching your back, contracting the lats to the max. Lower the weight in a controlled manner and repeat.

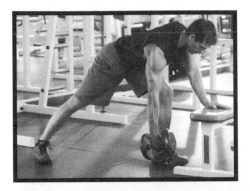

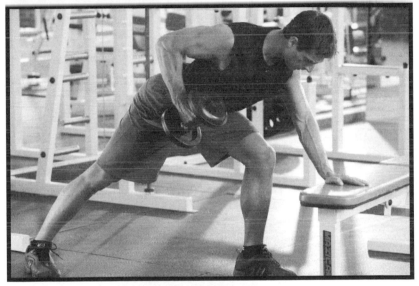

ONE-ARM ROW (ADVANCED)

Lean on your left hand and right leg and pull the weight with your right arm, as shown. With this particular back exercise you want to optimize the range of motion and stretch all the way down and pull the weight in the direction of your midsection. Again, in the process of pulling, try to arch the upper back for peak contraction. Use the heaviest weight possible with strict form. This exercise is great to develop your lats and will give thickness to your back.

Switch the weight to the left arm, change your legs to the opposite position, and do a set. Whatever stance you use, make sure your leaning arm and the opposite back leg both support the weight of your body. Keep going back and forth between arms.

Back CONCENTRATION EXERCISES

Lat Pulldown (wide grip)
Chinup or Gravetron-Supported Chinup
Vertical Pull Machine

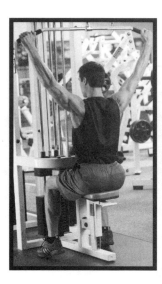 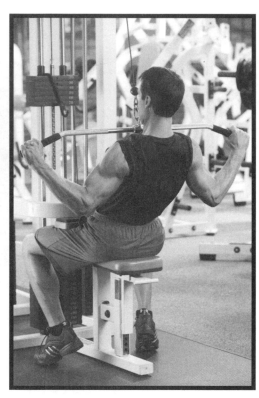

LAT PULLDOWN (WIDE GRIP)

When you choose this exercise as your second one, make sure that when you lean back, you execute the exercise the same way as the Lying T-Bar Machine—meaning that with every rep you extend your arms and keep the contraction on your lats. Don't stretch out your lats and shoulders by moving forward to the starting position.

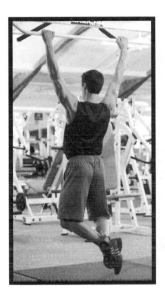

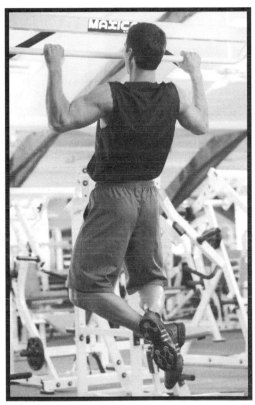

CHINUP OR
GRAVETRON-SUPPORTED CHINUP

If you cannot do at least 12 chinups, use the Gravetron instead. As you pull yourself up, try to increase the arch in your back instead of curling up. Pull your body up until the bar touches the middle of your chest, not your chin. Descend in a controlled manner until your arms are fully extended. Again, just like in the Lat Pulldown (wide grip), keep the shoulder area tight and your lats contracted.

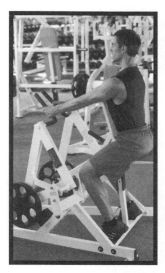
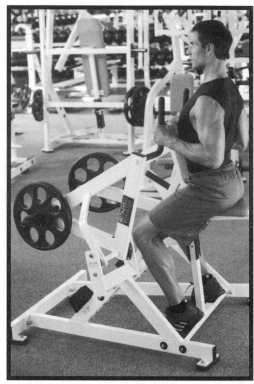

VERTICAL PULL MACHINE

This machine, when properly used, is the safest. It's used for one of the best exercises to focus on your lats. You can do the wide grip and put more emphasis on the outer parts of your lats, rear and middle delts, and upper traps (narrow reversed grip) or the narrow grip and put more emphasis on the whole lat area and lower traps. For instance, do as a basic exercise the Pulldown (narrow reversed grip), followed by the wide-grip Vertical Pull Machine. Or do as a basic exercise the Pulldown (medium grip), followed by the narrow-grip Vertical Pull Machine.

Square up with your shoulders and make sure your back is straight with a basic contraction of your lats. Don't hunch over; don't fully extend your back. Extend your elbows and start moving your shoulders backward with the help of your lats, then pull with your arms (just like the Low-Pulley Rows). Squeeze the muscle harder and harder, but don't yank the weight back. As you move forward again, control the weight—don't just drop it down. Remember the rule: 1 second on the pull part and 2 seconds on the release part.

Back ISOLATION EXERCISES

Cable-Cross Pulldown
Lat Flex

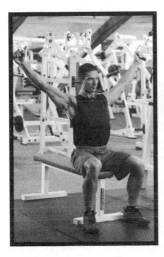
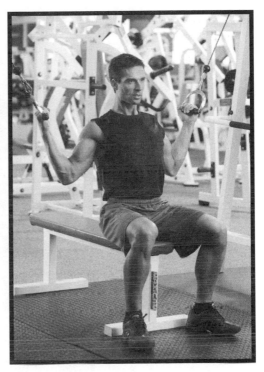

CABLE-CROSS PULLDOWN

This is the exercise that all my clients like, especially if you're looking for that pump at the end of a workout. It works the lats, lower traps, and all the smaller muscles around the shoulder blades. When you start the exercise, make sure your arms are fully extended, but keep the contraction on your lats so that your shoulders don't go up to your ears. Keep the back straight and pull down. As you pull down, arch your back and keep the emphasis on pulling through your lats. Don't try to pull the handles in front of your body. Your turning point comes when your hands reach shoulder level. Contract all the muscles in the back and let the hands go back up again.

Remember: Don't fully relax when your arms are extended, and don't let your shoulders travel up to your ears.

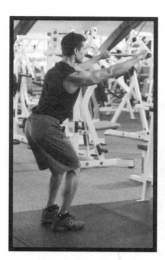

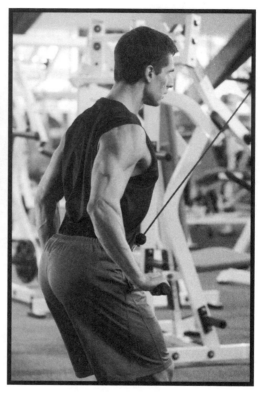

LAT FLEX

This exercise is great for your outer lats, of course, and if you do it the way I explain, it'll also work the lower traps and the entire latissimus dorsi area. Bend your knees and keep your back straight. Hold the bar with your hands about 15 to 20 inches apart, just a little wider than shoulder width. Keep your arms slightly bent, pointing the elbows out, and don't change the position. Move the weight halfway down, then move it toward your body; it's like a half-circle from top to bottom. You'll reach and maybe touch the tops of the quads (the front thigh muscles). Make sure that in the process of pulling the bar back you keep arching your back and shrugging your shoulder blades downward and together.

Biceps BASIC EXERCISES

E-Z Barbell Curl
Basic Straight Barbell Curl
Alternating Dumbbell Curl

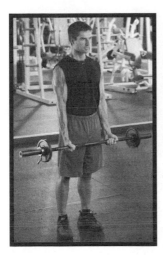
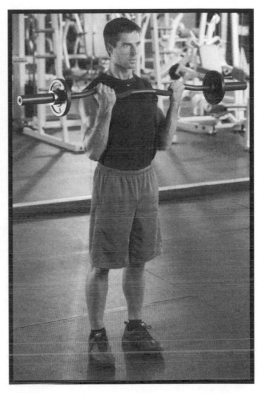

E-Z BARBELL CURL

One of the safest and most basic and effective biceps exercises is this E-Z Barbell Curl. Make sure in positioning yourself that your feet are at shoulder width, knees slightly bent, while contracting and squeezing quads, butt, and abs to stabilize the spine and to prevent yourself from cheating. While moving the weight up, squeeze and contract your lats. Keep your elbows close to your upper torso. Make sure that the wrist joint doesn't move back and forth; keep it in a neutral position. Keep moving the weight up until you've reached your clavicle (collarbone). Make a final squeeze with the biceps before letting the weight go down.

Remember: Don't drop the weight down—resist all the way down and even at the bottom, keeping the biceps in control of the movement by contracting the muscles. Repeat.

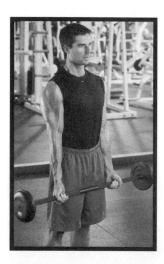

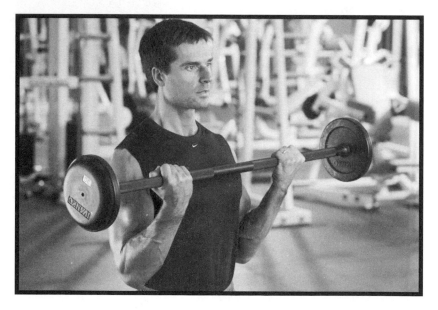

BASIC STRAIGHT BARBELL CURL

Perform the same as the E-Z Barbell Curl. When you pack on the weight, though, don't do any fewer than 12 reps in your 85 to 95 percent capacity range. The only problem I have with this particular exercise is that it poses more of a strain on the wrist joint. But make no mistake about it: It works the biceps.

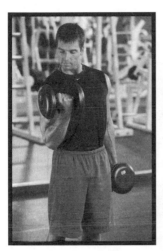

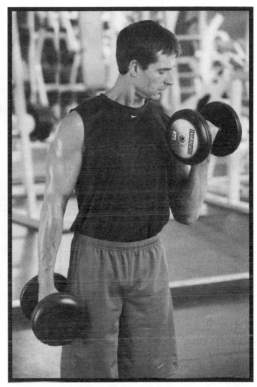

ALTERNATING DUMBBELL CURL

Using dumbbells on this exercise will put the focus per rep on the individual biceps. The stance remains the same as for the previous curls, but start with your hands down at your sides and your palms facing your body. Recently, I've noticed that when the palms are up throughout the upward and downward movement, you create a much more intense workload on the biceps, as long as the muscle stays contracted throughout the movement.

Biceps

CONCENTRATION/ISOLATION EXERCISES

Speedy Alternating Dumbbells
Straight Barbell Curl
Preacher Curl (advanced)
Cable Biceps Curl (advanced)

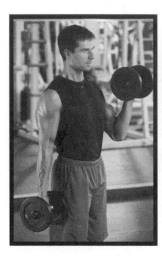
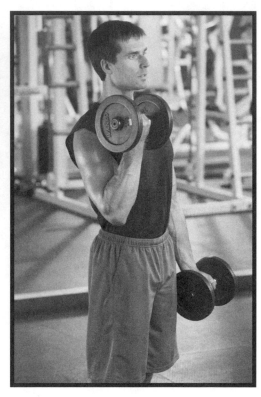

SPEEDY ALTERNATING DUMBBELLS

If you worked your biceps properly in the first part of your biceps workout, you will experience an unbelievable pump with this exercise. Speedy Alternating Dumbbells is a variation on the dumbbell curls. Keep your palms up while holding the dumbbells and alternate the dumbbells going up and down. While one dumbbell is being raised, the other is being lowered at the same pace. Don't pause at all, except at the end of the set.

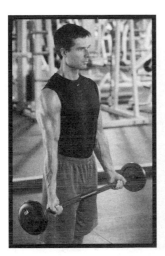

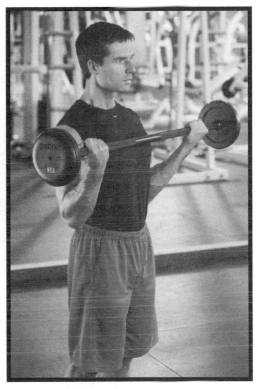

STRAIGHT BARBELL CURL

This is just like the Basic Straight Barbell Curls discussed earlier, only with less weight, higher reps, and a slightly wider grip than shoulder width.

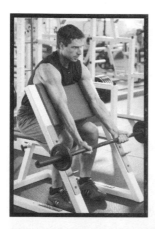

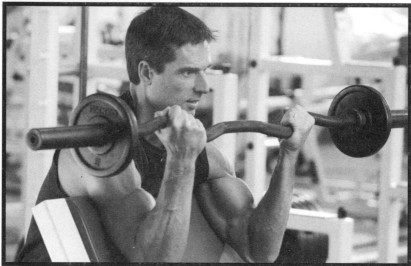

PREACHER CURL (ADVANCED)

Because of the isolated nature of this exercise, it's not recommended that you do this at the beginning of your Action Hero biceps workout. Nevertheless, after a couple of months of solid training, you can incorporate this exercise into your biceps routine. Make sure that your elbows are aligned with your shoulders and that you execute the fullest range of motion possible with the biceps: full extension of the arm while keeping the tension on the biceps muscles on the downward motion and full contraction on the upward motion. Make sure your shoulders stay down instead of moving up toward your ears. To keep your form perfect, you can also perform a machine version of this exercise.

Tip: Keep your lats contracted throughout the movement.

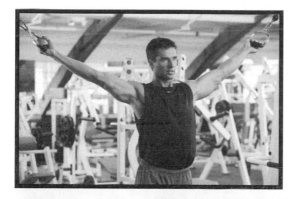

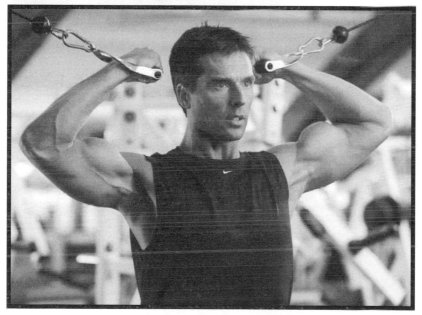

CABLE BICEPS CURL (ADVANCED)

With this one it's all about body control. You probably won't feel much on the first 10 reps. You might be tempted to move up in weight. But wait. As soon as you reach rep 11 with perfect form, it'll start to burn those biceps. It's a tricky one. Why is it all about body control? Because you have to lock up your body as you execute the exercise, as you did in the E-Z Barbell Curls. The only joints that are moving in this exercise are your elbows. Keep your elbows at ear level and curl the handles toward the sides of your head. Don't move the elbows forward; that's cheating.

Shoulders BASIC EXERCISES

Shoulder Press Machine
Seated or Standing Dumbbell Press
Front Press on Smith Machine

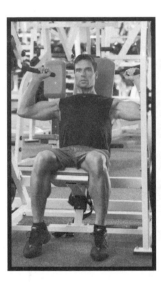
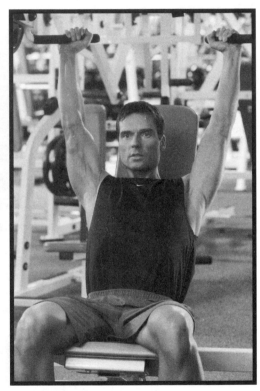

SHOULDER PRESS MACHINE

With the Shoulder Press Machine, you must find your own groove and hand position. Usually there are two grips: narrow and wide. Start by putting the bar or handles at ear level, pushing the weight up, and fully straightening your arms. Lower the weight in a controlled manner and make sure—this is very important in any shoulder press movement—that you keep your feet firmly on the ground, your back straight, your chest up, chin down, and that you look straight forward, as if you were saluting a general in the army.

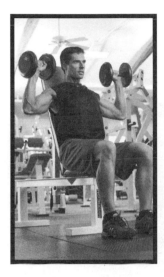
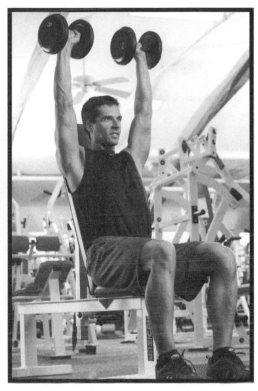

SEATED OR STANDING DUMBBELL PRESS

Make sure that your body is secure and steady. In a seated position, apply the same guidelines as for the previous exercise. With the Standing Dumbbell Press, put one foot in front of the other and keep your legs stable by contracting the quads and butt muscles. Keep your abs contracted and your back straight, chest up, and chin down. When executing the Dumbbell Press, whether seated or standing, make sure you press straight overhead, with roughly 4 inches between the two dumbbells. Lower the weights to about ear level. Balance the weights over your elbows so that they don't fall either outward, away from you, or inward, toward you. Keep your forearms perpendicular to the floor.

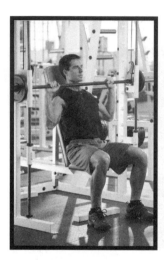

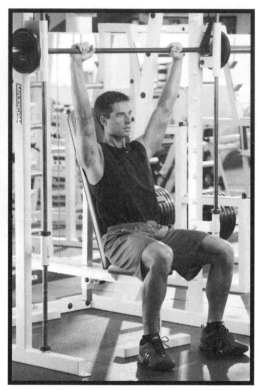

FRONT PRESS ON SMITH MACHINE

Put the bench on a sharp incline, almost straight. Leave enough space between your head and the bar to be able to pull it down as far as your Adam's apple. This exercise is a simplified version of the Seated Dumbbell Press.

Shoulders

CONCENTRATION EXERCISES

Upright Dumbbell Row
Upright Row (straight bar/cable)
Seated Bent-Over Laterals with Dumbbells
Rear Deltoids with Cables
Rear Deltoids on Fly/Rear Deltoids Machine

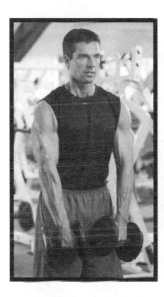
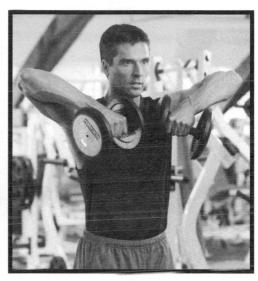

UPRIGHT DUMBBELL ROW

I like this exercise because it gives you lots of mobility, and you can adjust your hand position as you pull the weights from in front of your pelvis all the way to your clavicle. Never pull them beyond that, because you can pinch nerves in your neck and shoulder blade area. Stand erect with your legs slightly bent, squeeze your butt muscles and abs, and try to keep your upper body straight, even when you lower the weights from the highest point of the exercise. Make sure as you pull the weights up that you lead the movement with your elbows.

UPRIGHT ROW (STRAIGHT BAR/CABLE)
(NOT SHOWN)

Same principle as with the dumbbells, except that you're more constricted with your hands, so I advise caution by using a lighter weight and doing no fewer than 12 reps.

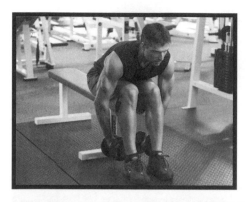

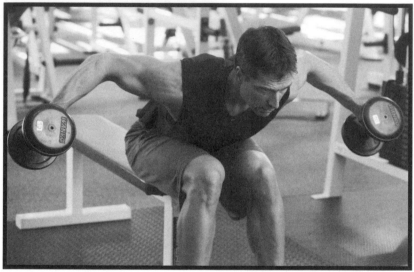

SEATED BENT-OVER LATERALS WITH DUMBBELLS

This is an excellent heavy-duty exercise. Sit on the edge of a flat bench and lean your chest on your quads. Make sure your spine stays straight; don't hunch over. Keep your arms slightly bent, even as you raise them sideways. As you raise the weights, arch your back but don't lift your chest off your quads; just arch your spine by contracting your lats and the rear delts and middle trapezius.

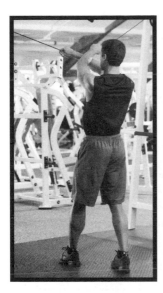
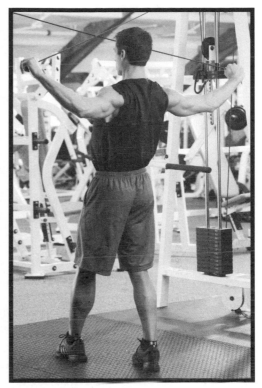

REAR DELTOIDS WITH CABLES

This is an exercise that targets the rear delts so specifically that you have to start out with a light weight, as low as 10 to 15 pounds on each side. Use a double-cable pulley. Lean against the weight and remain that way for the duration of the set. No swaying back and forth as you do this particular exercise. I always say, "You're like a rock in the waves; unmovable." Disconnect the handles, cross the cables, and hold them with your hands at the ends of the cables.

Your starting point is with straight, crossed-over arms. As you pull backward, bend them ever so slightly. Make sure you keep arching your back in the process of pulling the cables. Contract *all* the muscles in your back, especially the ones in the upper region, such as your rear delts, rhomboids, lower and middle traps, and even your big lats. It's a tough one to master, but once you have, you won't want to do anything else.

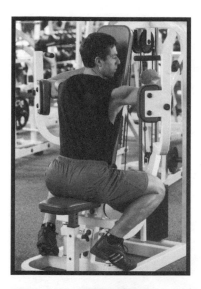

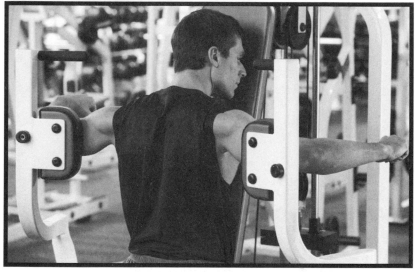

REAR DELTOIDS ON FLY/REAR DELTOIDS MACHINE

Probably the easiest exercise to train your rear delts, because you're basically guided through the exercise. Make sure, though, that you keep your back and spine straight, your head level and looking forward, and your arms slightly bent, and that you don't hunch as you pull the handles back.

Shoulders ISOLATION EXERCISES

Side Laterals (dumbbells or cables)
Front Laterals (dumbbells or cables)

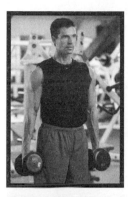

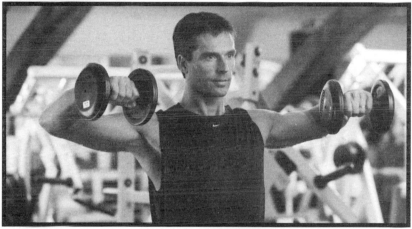

SIDE LATERALS (WITH DUMBBELLS)

Side Laterals, performed with either dumbbells or cables, probably the most rewarding exercise in the gym, at least as it relates to the burn and the pump. This is especially true when you finish off an Action Hero delt routine with the Side Laterals variation described here.

Make sure the dumbbells are on each side and that your body is as straight as can be: Keep your chest up, spine erect, and head straight. As you start moving the weight up, bend your elbows to a 90-degree angle between your forearm and upper arms. Never go higher than shoulder level with your arms; your traps start to help out in the exercise and your neck can be strained this way. As you move the weight down, extend your arms along your body again. Keep your body straight; don't collapse as you lower the weight.

SIDE LATERALS (WITH CABLES)

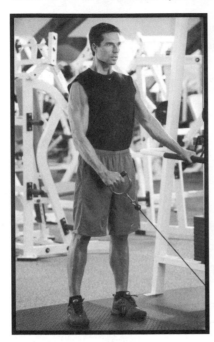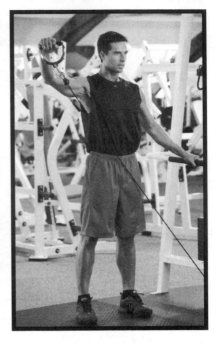

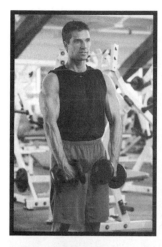

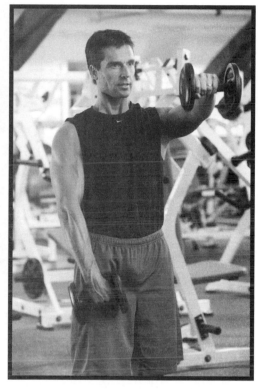

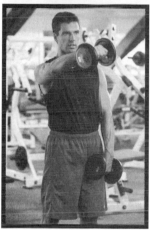

FRONT LATERALS (WITH DUMBBELLS)

Front Laterals, performed with either dumbbells or cables, goes perfectly with the heavy-load exercises such as the Seated Dumbbell Press and Upright Row. Stand erect with your knees ever so slightly bent. When you use the dumbbells, start right in front of your quads; when you use the cables, start next to your quads. With both exercises, move the weight in a circular movement upward to about forehead level. Resist the weight on the way down. Although it's okay to maintain a decent pace on the up and down movement, make sure you never lose control over the exercise and start to do a yo-yo movement up and down.

Tip: You can alternate Side Laterals and Front Laterals from one shoulder workout to the next.

FRONT LATERALS (WITH CABLES)

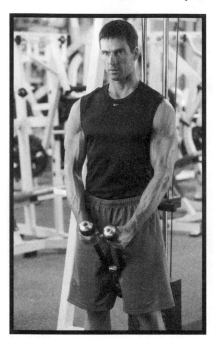 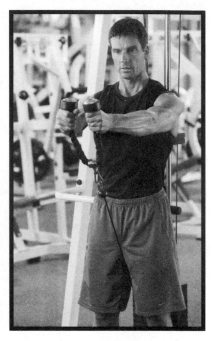

Legs BASIC EXERCISES

Leg Press
Squat
Dumbbell Squat
Stiff-Legged Deadlift

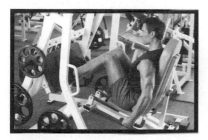

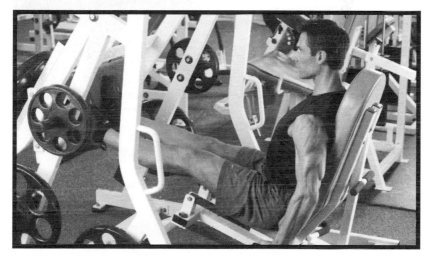

LEG PRESS

Leg presses are excellent for building strong, muscular legs. Even though squats are considered the best leg builder of them all, I prefer to recommend this exercise to my clients. Position yourself on the machine and, as you release the levers that hold the platform that you're pressing your feet against, make sure your lower back is flat. Control the weight by contracting your quads and butt muscles, and start arching your lower back, making sure it doesn't come off the machine. Lower the weight according to the "elevator principle" (no yo-yos here, either). Resist. . . . As your quads touch your rib cage, push back up. When you extend and lock your knees, do it gently and keep your muscles contracted.

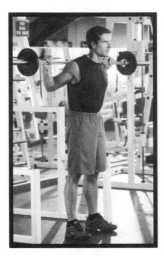
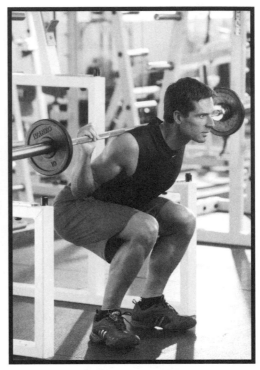

SQUAT

Every Stage Three athlete should know how to do squats. This exercise will give you the leg strength, overall body strength, coordination, balance, and ultimately the AH physique that you've been dreaming about. As you take the weight off the rack, be aware of it. Contract every fiber in your body to control the weight on your shoulders, not your neck. Maintain an erect body position when descending; leaning too far forward can put unnecessary strain on your lower back. Foot spacing is a personal thing, but usually keeping the feet shoulder width apart works for most athletes. Lower the weight until the tops of your quads are parallel to the floor. On the way up, make sure you keep your body erect, squeezing your quads and glutes simultaneously.

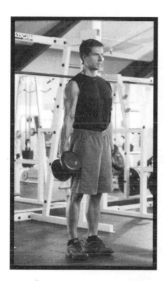
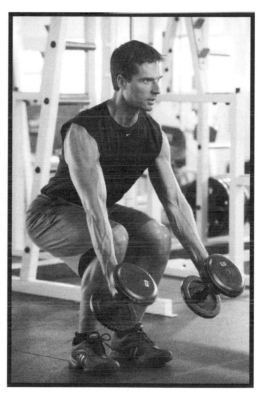

DUMBBELL SQUAT

Stand erect with feet shoulder width apart and one dumbbell of equal weight in each hand. Keep the dumbbells at the sides of your body and don't let them drift to the center of your body. Use the same technique as in the regular Squat.

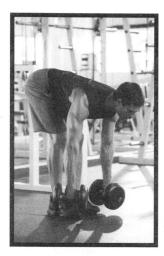
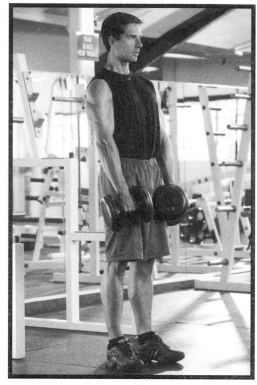

STIFF-LEGGED DEADLIFT

The Stiff-Legged Deadlift shouldn't be done with completely straight legs. A slight bend in the knees should always be present. You can do this exercise with dumbbells or with a straight bar. Personally, I like the dumbbells better, because they offer more mobility, and you can adjust the hand position according to your preference without compromising the exercise's effectiveness.

Start from the floor and lift the weight up first as though you were doing a squat (bending the knees, keeping the head up and back arched). As you start downward with the weight, keep it close to your body. As you continue to go down, keep the weight close to your legs. Keep your knees slightly bent, and put most of the pressure on the heel of your foot. Arch your back and keep your head up. As you start back up, make sure you keep your knees bent and let your hamstrings and butt muscles do the work. Again, keep the weight close to your body. As you stand tall and erect, squeeze your quads and butt muscles without shifting your pelvis forward. Tuck your butt underneath your spine and pelvis.

Legs CONCENTRATION EXERCISES

Sissy Squat
Lying/Seated Leg Curl
One-Legged Skater Lunge (on bench)
Cross-Step Lunge
Lunge on Smith Machine

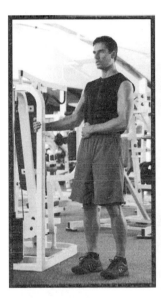
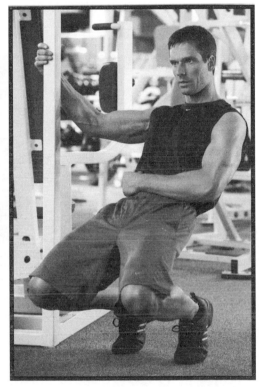

SISSY SQUAT

There's a misconception that this exercise is too hard on the knees. This is only the case when it's performed incorrectly or when too much emphasis is put on the quads.

Position your feet shoulder width apart. At the top of the movement, stand completely straight with knees locked, the quads completely flexed in conjunction with the butt muscles. At this point, you're leaning slightly backward so your body is at a 75-degree angle. As you go down, bend your knees, bend your hips, and lean forward, taking pressure away from the knees. Never lose control when you go down; always feel the contraction of the muscles in your quads and butt. Your body should move like an accordion.

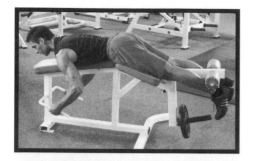

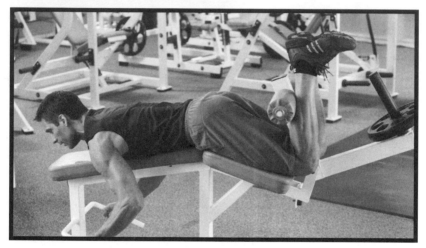

LYING LEG CURL

Either of these two exercises is a great hamstring developer. It works all three parts of the hamstrings.

The Lying Leg Curl is somewhat self-explanatory, but remember to always push your pelvis down and keep your abs and butt muscles contracted so that you don't arch and strain your lower back. Lie on the bench and curl the weight up. Keep your feet neutral—don't flex your calves, but fully isolate the hamstrings. Think about curling a weight up with your arms, as you do with barbell biceps curls. Squeeze the hamstrings until you reach the top, then slowly release the muscles and go down again. Don't drop the weight. As you come down to a full extension of the knees again, repeat the movement.

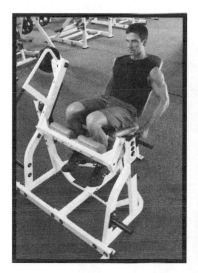
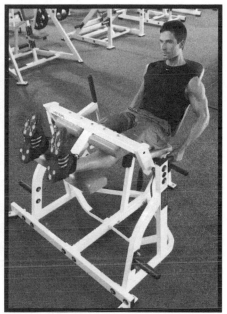

SEATED LEG CURL

For the Seated Leg Curl, get on the machine and brace yourself by squeezing your abs to protect your lower back, then push with your hands against the machine. This will help protect your body from moving back and forth on the machine.

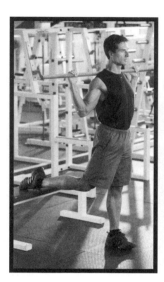
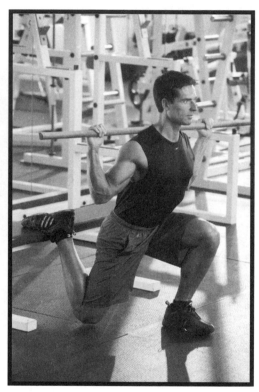

ONE-LEGGED SKATER LUNGE (ON BENCH)

This particular exercise really isolates the butt and quad area. However, be warned: If you do this exercise the wrong way, you'll fall over. Put one foot on a bench and the other about 2 to 3 feet away from the bench (the distance depends on the length of your legs). Go down slowly, like you do with any other squat movement. Keep your head and chest up, arch your back, and let your body move down like a skier going off a ski slope. Keep the pressure predominantly on the heel of your foot. Go back up and stand completely upright, straightening the knee and hip joint (and squeezing the quads and butt muscles). Complete all reps on one leg, then switch legs.

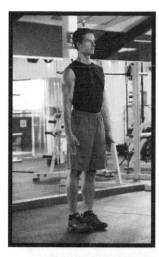

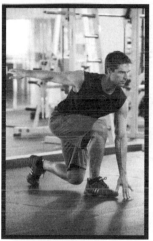

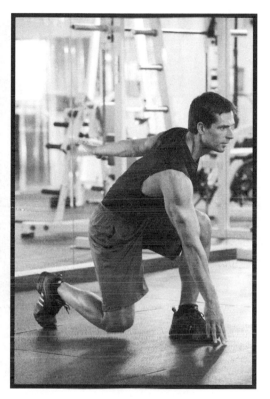

CROSS-STEP LUNGE

Just like in the previous exercise, there's a lot of balance involved and ultimate isolation of the quads and glutes. Yet, this is one of the best leg exercises around. As you step forward, make sure you make a soft landing on the heel of the foot, and go down until you touch the ground with the knee of the leg that's in the back. While you're going down, reach with the opposite hand in front of the leg that you stepped out with. Push off in a straight upward line and repeat with the other leg and hand. Always keep your back straight, even though you reach forward with your hand. Just make sure that you bend your knees enough so you can actually touch the foot that's in front of you.

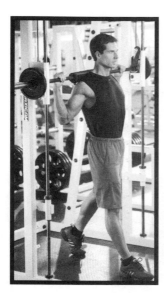
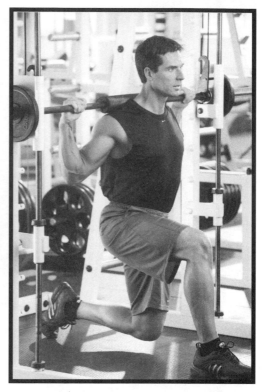

LUNGE ON SMITH MACHINE

Lunges are great for working the quads and glutes simultaneously. They are one of the most exhausting exercises there are, since you have to alternate your two legs without too much rest between each one.

Get the bar securely positioned on your shoulders, and put one foot forward about 2 feet in front of you (this is the leg you'll be working). The other foot should be placed about 2 feet behind you. Unlock the machine and descend in a controlled manner. Make sure you bend the knee of the front leg just as much as you bend your hip joint. That way you'll go down in a straight line until you touch the floor with the knee of the leg that's behind you. Arch your back as you go down, and make sure you keep your head straight.

On the way up, extend the knee at the same pace as you extend the hip. At the top of the movement, completely flex your back leg, so you can squeeze the muscles of both legs as well as your butt muscles.

Legs ISOLATION EXERCISES

Leg Extension
Butt Squeeze

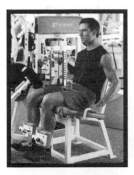

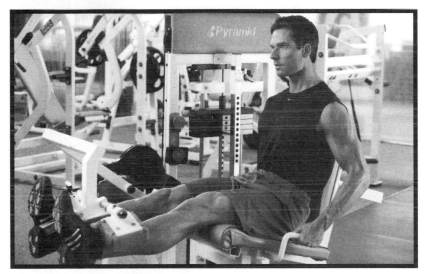

LEG EXTENSION

This is a great exercise that isolates the quads. Finish your workout with a couple sets of Leg Extensions, and you'll have that sought-after pump. Even though the exercise is somewhat self-explanatory, you want to make sure you don't try to go all the way up (hyperextend). Follow the movement of the exercise until you extend your knees, and then, at the top of the exercise, push your feet away as if you were trying to push against something right in front of you with your feet. As you reach the down part of the exercise, don't lose complete contraction of the muscles. Go down until your upper leg is at a 90-degree angle to your lower leg. Then repeat the movement.

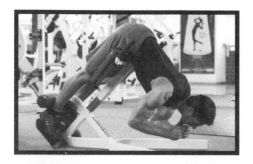

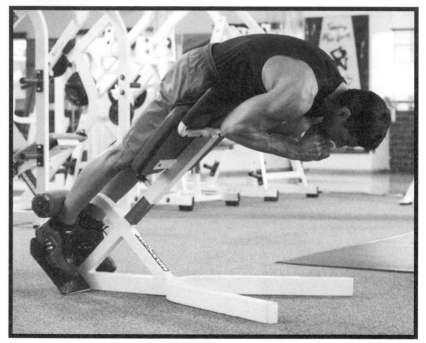

BUTT SQUEEZE

This exercise really targets and isolates the butt muscles. Get on a hyperextension machine and hang all the way down, even slightly arching your back. As you come up with your body, initiate the movement by contracting your glutes. As you move up, contract your abs, bringing your chin to your chest. Crunch your body, putting the maximum contraction on your glutes and abs. Slowly release, and go back down in a controlled manner.

The "Other" Muscle Groups: Abs, Calves, and Forearms

I don't train abs, calves, and forearms like other muscle groups. Yes, they're probably the most exposed of all the groups, especially during the summer months. But most people can't train them effectively without wasting a lot of energy and time. That's why I suggest you train them after your regular Action Hero workout, and after your aerobic activity.

When training abs, calves, and forearms, the workout typically should take less than 20 minutes. But the sets are long, the rests short, and the exercises challenging.

Let's start with abs. The first routine is good for beginners (Stage One) getting used to training their abs. Even when you're an intermediate (Stage Two) or advanced (Stage Three) athlete, with the right number of reps and short resting time, this routine will deliver a good overall abs workout. The second abs routine (on page 168) is more advanced.

Abs 1

Crunch
Side-to-Side
Knee Lift
Rocky's

Make a fist with your hand. Now squeeze tight and release, squeeze tight and release ever so slightly. This is the same type of muscle contraction you want to use when training your abs—never let go of that first initial contraction. Not only is this a safer way to train your abs, it's also more effective, because you never relax the muscles at any point; therefore, your abs never have time to recover.

The abdominals are a very resilient muscle group. They're exposed to muscle strain all day, and they're used to a lot of muscle contraction. Think about it: They help you balance while playing sports, running, walking, even sitting down. So if you really want to develop these muscles, you must create that extra dimension of additional workload. The secret is to train them correctly.

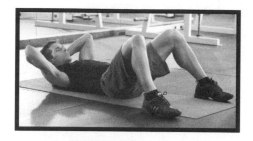

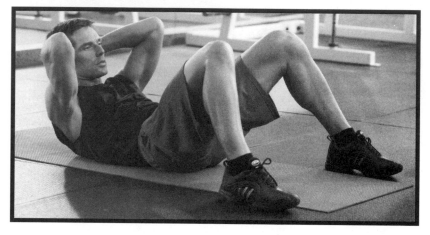

CRUNCH

You may have heard that crunches are dangerous for your neck or that when you do them you won't even feel the burn in your abdominal muscles. Here's how to do them correctly.

Lie on a mat, bend your knees, and put one foot on each side of the mat. Either place your hands across your chest, interlock your fingers behind your head, or reach between your legs. Always make sure that you keep the muscles in the front of your neck contracted; you don't want your head to fall backward.

Before you even start thinking about crunching your upper torso (*not* yanking on your head), make sure you push your lower back against the mat. This will engage your abdominals even before starting the exercise. Dig your feet into the floor and now start crunching your body. Don't come up all the way—that's not a crunch; that's a complete situp—but instead squeeze the abs, just like you would if you made a strong fist. On the way back, try to maintain the contraction on your abs and lower your torso to just before you hit your shoulder blades on the mat. Do 15 or 20 reps in the beginning. Work up to 30 or even 40.

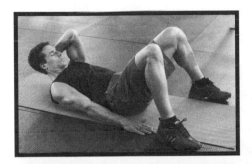

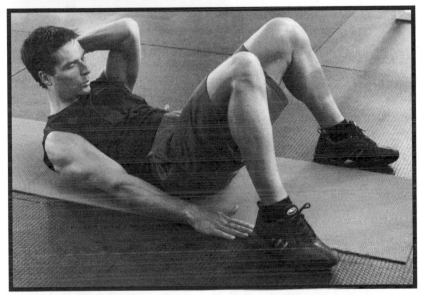

SIDE-TO-SIDE

This exercise is a variation of the regular crunches—you leave one hand behind your neck and put the other next to your body. Crunch your upper torso just like in the regular crunches, but this time take your elbow right to the center of your body (the crotch). Don't reach for your knees or the opposing leg. It's more of a circular movement. Do 15 to 20 reps on each side.

Tip: Can you figure out how many reps of an abs exercise are good for you? Take it easy in the beginning. The gauge by which you should determine number of reps is the discomfort you feel in your abdominal region. After a few weeks, you can apply what I call the golden rule: When your abs start to burn, and I mean *really* burn, count 10 more reps. Now you can always tell how many reps are good for you—10 more after the burn for that particular abs routine on that particular day.

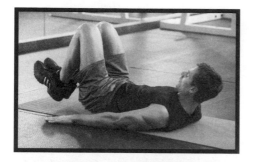

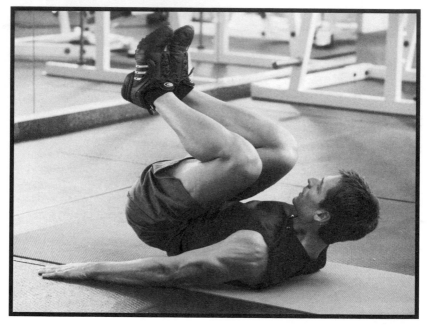

KNEE LIFT

Stay on your back, put your legs together, and bend your knees at a 90-degree angle. Keep both hands next to your body and raise, or roll, your knees up. Don't jerk up, but gradually start moving up until your knees are in front of your chest. You may even lift your hips off the ground. Push your hands hard against the floor; it really helps to keep the focus on your abs and control the exercise. On your way down, control the weight of your legs and softly touch the floor with your heels. Repeat.

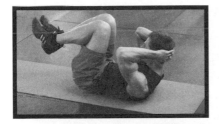
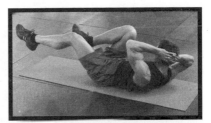

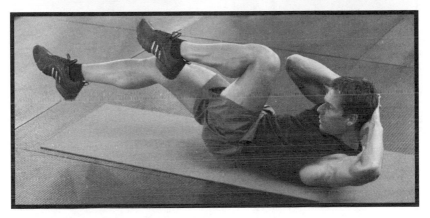

ROCKY'S

This is one of the single most valuable exercises there is, if done correctly—not just to get razor-sharp abs but also to create mobility and strength throughout the hip and lower back joints.

Stay on your back, leaving your feet on the floor as you do when performing a crunch. Then crunch up your upper torso without pulling your head. While keeping the contraction on your abs, lift up both legs. Your abs are fully contracted now, like that fist that I talked about earlier. Slowly move your left elbow to your right knee. Try to bring the elbow to the knee and the knee to the elbow: They're almost meeting each other. Do the same for the other side and repeat. Make sure that your shoulder blades don't touch the mat and that you don't strain your lower back. Now start alternating at a higher pace: left, right, left, right.

Abs 2

Hanging Leg Raise
Army-Style Situp
Bench Knee Lift
Bench Crunch
Rocky's

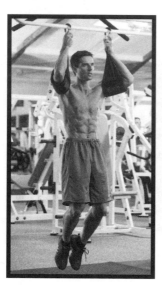
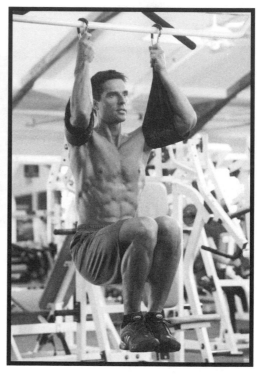

HANGING LEG RAISE

Place your arms in the chin rack with the soft, padded arm slings. Hold the top of the slings with your hands. As you hang, let your legs dangle with your abdominals tight, your quads slightly tightened. Bring your knees up in the direction of your nose. Curl your body up, aiming for your nose with your knees. On the way down make sure you resist. When you reach the point where your legs are fully extended, continue the exercise by quickly doing another repetition. With this exercise it's more effective to keep going. Keep up the momentum. Work up to 20 to 30 reps. If you want a more intense workout, hang on to a wide-grip chin bar and do the same exercise. Do roughly one to two sets of 15 to 30 reps, depending on your fitness level.

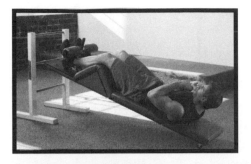

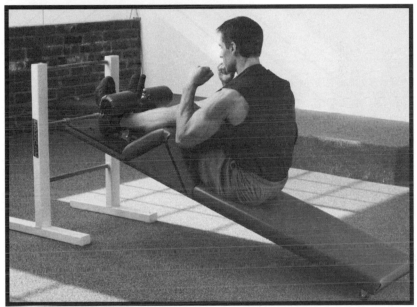

ARMY-STYLE SITUP

This is an advanced yet safe exercise, as long as you contract your abdominal region at all times, during the ascending and descending parts of the exercise. The trick is to hook your feet under the bench and start contracting your abdominals even before you start the exercise. Keep squeezing your abs and make your way up to where your chest touches your quads. Contract your abs harder at the top. Roll your body back down to the bench, but keep the abs contracted. Never let go! Repeat. Do one to two sets of 20 to 40 reps.

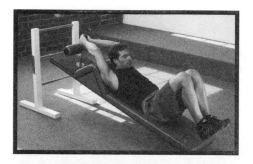

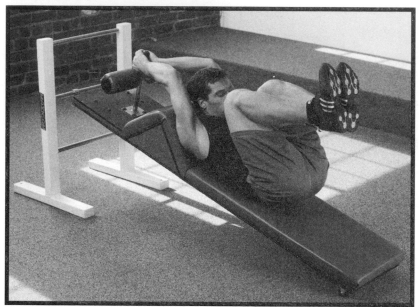

BENCH KNEE LIFT

These are the same as the Knee Lifts on the mat explained in Abs 1, except they're done on a bench. This time, however, hold on tight to the bench. Keep your legs bent, and bring up your knees while holding on even tighter to the bench, as if you were bringing your hands toward your knees. On the way down, pass the edge of the bench and touch the floor. Make sure you have full control of your abs and that you don't put any unnecessary strain on your lower back. This exercise is very advanced, and if you have trouble, you shouldn't go past the edge of the bench. Work your way up to one to two sets of 15 to 20 reps.

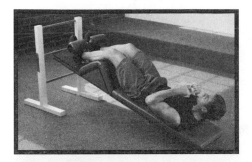

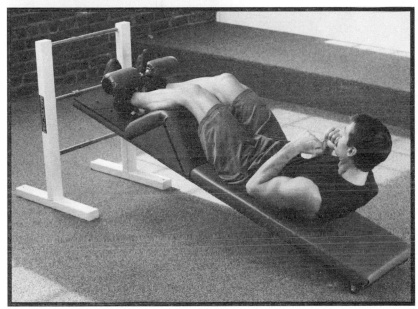

BENCH CRUNCH

Use the same bench again. Turn yourself around to the same position as for the Army-Style Situps. This time don't go all the way up, but do crunches. To increase the level of difficulty, vary the position of the bench, inclining it so that your legs are a little higher than your head. Make sure in this position that you really push your lower back into the bench by putting that initial contraction on the abs before even starting the exercise. Work yourself up to one to two sets of 40 reps.

ROCKY'S

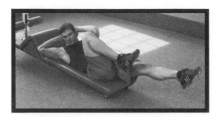

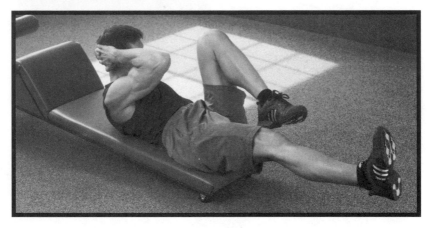

Finish with the Rocky's for the ultimate and extreme burn. Do as many reps as possible.

TRAINING ABS SAFELY

There are a million other exercises, and I encourage you to try new ones, but not before you understand the basic principles of training your abdominal muscles. Here are the main points to keep in mind.

- Be aware of your abs before you start your exercise. Contract them in anticipation of the exercise.

- Remember to push your lower back against the floor or bench.

- Never let go of the contraction.

- Never hyperextend your back. Stay crunched through the motion, even on the way down.

- Keep the abs in control of the movement at all times.

- Squeeze your abs as though you were squeezing your hand into a fist.

If there's a strain in your lower back at any point during any of the more advanced abs exercises, go back to Abs 1. If there's a consistent ache, especially in your spine, have a professional check it out. Sometimes as you do your exercise, you might feel a burning sensation on each side of your spine. Usually, that's an indication that you're not squeezing your abs hard enough and that you're arching your back (not crunching). Your lower back muscles are tensing up, even to the point of a muscle spasm. Just back off for a minute before continuing the exercise. Eventually, your abdominal muscles will strengthen to the point where they can compensate for the back strain.

Calves

Standing Calf Raise
Seated Calf Raise
Alternate Standing Calf Raise

If you have well-developed calves, you have them. If you don't, you don't. You can train all you want and try the most advanced and latest calf routines, but if you don't have the genetic makeup for long, diamond-shaped calves, you'll probably never get the calves that you want.

Nevertheless, you can always improve your calves by making them stronger and bigger.

Calves are easy to train: It takes short workouts, high reps, and short breaks between sets, using a heavy weight. Calf muscles are strong and can endure a lot of pressure. In the beginning of your calves routine, however, use only your body weight with the standing calf raises, and do 10 reps per set. See how they're doing the next day. Add a few more reps, a few more sets, and increase the weight gradually. Once they're used to training, blast them. Just like abs, you can train them quite frequently; every other day is fine.

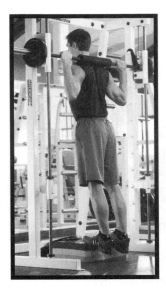
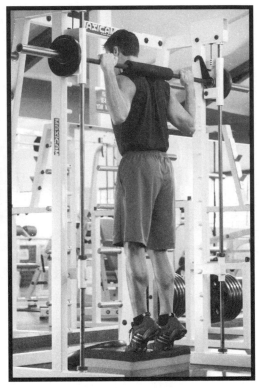

STANDING CALF RAISE

Get yourself under the Standing Calf Raise machine and lift the weight with your legs. Squat and push the pads up. Keep your knees slightly bent, not fully extended, and push off with your toes. On the way down, make sure you resist the weight, and don't make any bouncy movements; you can inflict severe injuries to your Achilles tendons.

Because this muscle group responds quickly, you have to train it with high reps (roughly 15 to 20) and short breaks (20 seconds or so). Use quite a bit of weight on this particular exercise—150 to 500 pounds or even more for advanced Action Hero fanatics.

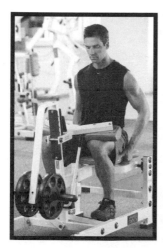
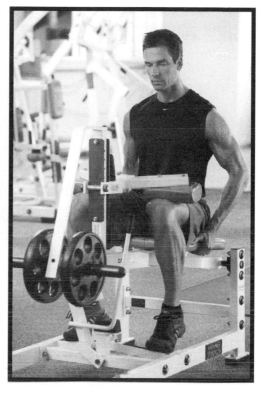

SEATED CALF RAISE

This particular exercise works the lower parts of the calf muscles. I like to do this exercise when I'm exhausted from the Standing Calf Raises. Execute two to three sets with a weight you can handle for at least 15 reps. Make sure that you're working hard and can feel the burn after about 10 reps, because you want to stay in the 85 to 95 percent range (HIS). As I warned you before, use extreme caution at the beginning of any calf routine. If you start out too intensely, you might not even be able to walk the next day. The pain will be excruciating. So limit your weight on the first day of your calf routine.

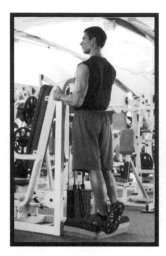

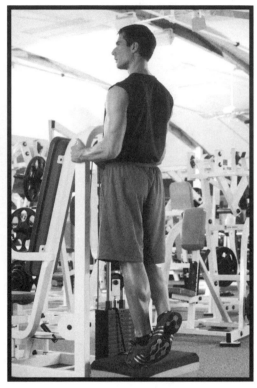

ALTERNATE STANDING CALF RAISE

This exercise is great to flush your calves with blood. Stand on one leg on a flat surface, and do a Calf Raise but without any weight, just your body weight. Do as many
reps as you can, up to 30. Switch calves and repeat. Do two sets with each calf.

Forearms

Wrist Curl (with rope)
Wrist Curl (on bench)

Well-developed forearms on men display strength and health and, to women, can even convey security. When you train according to the Action Hero training system, you work your forearms with almost every exercise. I haven't trained my forearms in 23 years. The same is true for my calves.

Just like with calves, if you are blessed with well-proportioned forearms and they're symmetrically developed compared to your upper arms, you have no business working them unless, of course, you want them to be even stronger. Maybe you want to make your grip on a tennis racquet more firm, or you want to make your wrist shot in ice hockey more powerful. For specific sports, you can always do a few forearm exercises that will make you even more powerful.

HOT OR COLD?

Most of us work out in air-conditioned gyms, but where's the all-important oxygen for a strenuous workout?

In my opinion, gym temperatures should be 72° to 75°F (humidity about 30 to 60 percent), with a mild airflow that can deliver a steady supply of oxygen. The trick is to adjust your workout to the weather. If the temperature outside is more than 80°, move at a slower pace, and take more frequent water breaks. If you find yourself running out of steam, stop and do some abdominal work or skip the cardio for that day. Let's be honest: Nothing in life is comfortable at 80°-plus.

On the other hand, if you have a problem with overheating because you're out of shape or overweight, ask someone to turn on the air-conditioning. In this scenario, it's more important to stay cool than to sweat profusely.

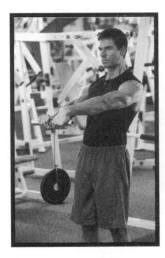
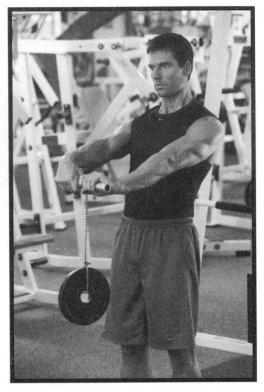

WRIST CURL (WITH ROPE)

Stand on a bench and hold the short bar in your hands at hip level. Alternately curl your wrists and flex your forearms. Keep curling until the weight on the rope reaches the bar. Either keep curling so the weight flips over onto the other side of the bar or just start curling the other way around so that the weight goes down again. Go easy the first couple of times. Do this exercise by itself using about 10 pounds of weight. Take a break after each round or just keep going.

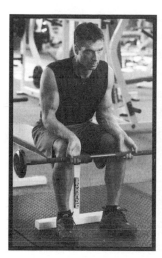
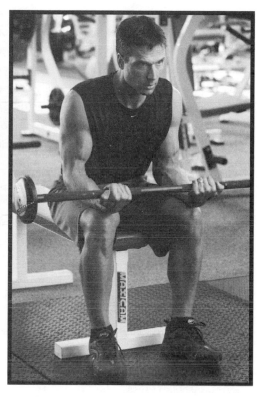

WRIST CURL (ON BENCH)

Sit on a bench and keep your wrists on the edges of your knees with your palms facing up. Hold the fixed-weight bar in your hands. Roll the bar all the way down to your fingers only to curl them back up and flex the wrist. Repeat. Do three to four sets of 15 reps.

Finally, do this same exercise with your palms facing down. Keep a tight squeeze on the bar and move your hands up and down. Again, try for three to four sets of 15 reps.

WHILE TRAVELING

For those of you who are constantly on the road—traveling to and from, staying in hotels—here's an Action Hero training system that works all the major muscle groups, stimulates bloodflow, and conditions your cardiovascular system.

Many of my high-profile clients, who travel the world and stay at every hotel imaginable, have found this system beneficial. You can alternate these workouts as you please. For maximum conditioning benefits, you should train no less than every 3 days while traveling. If possible, do an every-other-day cycle.

Where indicated, perform the exercises at 75 to 95 percent of your capacity. To do this, pick a weight that feels comfortable on the first set. Because you're doing multiple sets, fatigue will set in, and soon you'll experience an 85 to 95 percent effect on your muscles.

ROUTINE ONE	SETS	REPS	PERCENTAGE
7- to 10-minute bike ride or 5 minutes running in place			
Dumbbell Squat	4	20	75 to 95

Hold dumbbells on each side of the body as you go down—usually no more than 15 pounds per hand.

Superset w/

Stiff-Legged Deadlift	4	20	75 to 95

If you're new to my program, take no more than 10 pounds in each hand and go slowly on the descending part of the movement.

Superset w/

Standing Dumbbell Press	4	15	75 to 95

Superset w/

Any Barbell (or Dumbbell) Curl	3	15	75 to 95

Superset w/

Overhead Dumbbell Extension	3	15	75 to 95

As indicated, do all the exercises listed above in succession, then take a water break, followed by three more rounds on the leg and shoulder exercises and two more rounds on the arm exercises.

15-minute cardio test on a bike or 10 to 15 minutes running in place			
Rocky's	3	30–50	—

Note: Routine One and Routine Two are interchangeable.

ROUTINE TWO	SETS	REPS	PERCENTAGE
7- to 10-minute bike ride or 5 minutes running in place			
Pulldown (medium or reversed grip)	4	15	75 to 95
Superset w/			
Any kind of chest press (machine)	4	15	75 to 95
Superset w/			
Side Laterals	4	15	75 to 95
Superset w/			
Any Barbell (or Dumbbell) Curl	3	15	75 to 95
Superset w/			
Dippy	3	15	75 to 95

As indicated, do all exercises above in succession, then take a water break, followed by three more rounds on the back, chest, and shoulder exercises, and two more rounds on the arm exercises.

15-minute cardio test on a bike or 10 to 15 minutes running in place			
Rocky's	3	30–50	—

The Stages Programs

STAGE ONE

When you take it slow in the beginning of your Action Hero workout adventure, you'll enjoy a great feeling of mild fatigue right after your workouts, a great night's sleep, and a spiritual revival in the weeks to follow.

Stage One is a light-to-moderate training program built around your first several weeks. It includes 2 days of weight lifting and, depending on whether you want to lose weight as well as build muscle, 2 or 3 days of aerobic activity and 2 or 3 days of rest.

On weight-lifting days, begin by warming up for 10 minutes on your favorite cardio machine. The first several minutes will feel like a breeze. After the first 2 minutes, increase the intensity to a comfortable level. If you get winded, simply slow down until you regain your breath. Then pick up the pace again.

Let's say, for example, you've set your stationary bike at level 8 (a moderate-intensity level), and you're cruising at about 85 rpm. If this pace becomes uncomfortable, simply lower the level to 7 and reduce your speed to 75 rpm. Once you regain your strength, return to level 8 at 85 rpm. If you can sustain the pace this time, ride out the remainder of your 10 minutes. Otherwise, keep adjusting the level and pace down and up as you become winded and recover. After several days of training, you should be able to increase your intensity level.

After your warmup, do some mild stretching for 1 minute. Take a sip of water and a 1-minute break before you begin the weight-lifting part of your workout. If you feel good after three rounds and you think you can do more, go ahead and do as many as two more rounds—just don't increase the weight.

Take a look at the following weekly program for a 33-year-old man in average condition who wants to lose 20 pounds. He works at a sedentary job from nine to five, Monday through Friday. Does he sound like anyone you know?

Sunday: Aerobic activity for 20 to 60 minutes

Monday: Day One workout and 20 minutes of aerobic activity

Tuesday: Aerobic activity for 20 to 60 minutes

Wednesday: Rest

Thursday: Day Two workout and 20 minutes of aerobic activity

Friday: Aerobic activity for 20 to 60 minutes

Saturday: Rest

For those who don't want to lose any weight but would like to become stronger and healthier, here's a program that will work for you.

Sunday: Rest

Monday: Day One workout

Tuesday: Aerobic activity for 20 to 60 minutes

Wednesday: Rest

Thursday: Day Two workout

Friday: Aerobic activity for 20 to 60 minutes

Saturday: Rest

Keep in mind that if you follow either of these programs, your health will change for the better and you'll have more energy at work and play—even in bed! You'll probably notice improvements in your stamina and well-being after the first week. After 2 or 3 weeks, you'll have begun to lay the foundation for optimal health for the rest of your life. But you must follow the program carefully; otherwise, your foundation will crumble like a poorly constructed house.

Here are the specific exercises for workout days. As I said earlier, a superset is two or more exercises performed one after the other. These exercises typically work opposing muscles, such as back and chest or biceps and triceps, allowing you to work one muscle group while resting the other. (*Note:* Detailed descriptions of all these exercises appear in the "Body Sculpting" section, which starts on page 110.)

DAY ONE	SETS	REPS	PERCENTAGE
Pull Machine	3	12	50
Superset w/			
Vertical Bench Press Machine	3	12	50
Superset w/			
Upright Row	3	12	50
Superset w/			
E-Z Barbell Curl	3	12	50
Superset w/			
Triceps Pushdown	3	12	50

DAY TWO	SETS	REPS	PERCENTAGE
Lat Pulldown	3	12	50
Superset w/			
Incline Smith Machine Press	3	12	50
Superset w/			
Side Laterals	3	12	50
Superset w/			
Alternating Dumbbell Curl	3	12	50
Superset w/			
Dippy	3	12	50

If you feel good after three rounds on each of the two workout days, and you think you can do more rounds, go ahead and do as many as two more—just don't increase the weight. At least, not yet.

After your workout, do another 15 minutes of aerobic activity to boost your cardiovascular and respiratory systems. Choose between the treadmill and stationary bike.

The objective of this mild cardio test is to determine whether you can elevate your heart rate and sustain it without becoming winded. Keep in mind the following guidelines: If you've never done any serious exercising prior to your first workout, but your doctor has given you the go-ahead, keep your heart rate at around 50 percent of your cardiovascular capacity. If, however, you've been working out for a while at a heart rate of 65 to 80 percent capacity, but you're ready to move into the Action Hero program at full speed, then boost your heart rate within the first 2 minutes to as high as 80 percent capacity.

Here's how to determine your cardiovascular capacity: 220 − age = maximum heart rate. Fifty percent of your maximum heart rate equals 50 percent of your capacity. Eighty percent of your maximum heart rate equals 80 percent of your capacity. Voilà!

I'll often have a client exercise on a stationary bike set at level 8 at 90 rpm. If he can manage that without any noticeable strain, I'll raise the level to 9 and ask him to maintain the 90 rpm after the first minute.

If he's still doing well after yet another minute, I'll raise the level to 10 and have him continue for another 11 minutes or so. If, however, after a couple of minutes the intensity seems too high, I'll lower the level to 8 but maintain the speed for the first minute.

Once the client recovers his wind, I'll take it up again to level 10 and leave it there until he's pedaled for 11 minutes, then drop it back to levels 6 to 8 at 75 rpm for the cooldown phase.

To summarize, the cardio test breaks down as follows.

1 minute—level 8 at 90 rpm

1 minute—level 9 at 90 rpm

11 minutes—levels 8 to 10 at 90 rpm

2 minutes—levels 6 to 8 at 75 rpm

This is the foundation of every postworkout aerobic session. But, you're not finished just yet. Complete the workout with a few simple abdominal exercises (see the "Abs 1" section on page 163 for detailed descriptions): Crunches, Side-to-Sides, Knee Lifts, and Rocky's.

Begin with about 20 Crunches, 15 Side-to-Sides (on each side, of course), 20 Knee Lifts, and up to 30 Rocky's on each side. It's okay if you need to take breaks in the middle of your set, but try to complete all the reps in the set first. Then, take no longer than a 30-second break between sets.

On days when you don't work out with weights, get in some aerobic activity to stimulate optimal fat burning in your body. Figure on about 20 to 60 minutes, depending on your physical condition and goals. Don't worry about whether it's cardiovascular exercise, which conditions the heart and lungs for increased performance with endurance. Concentrate instead on bringing your heart rate up to 120 to 130 beats per minute.

A trick to increase your heart rate on the treadmill without running is to raise the runway's elevation. This also firms up your quads and glutes.

One of the best times for aerobic activity is in the morning before breakfast. If you must eat something first, have an apple with half a cup of coffee. That should get you going. It's even better to leave the apple out altogether because your body will start burning fat right away. And if you can stomach the coffee without the apple, you'll really be in business: Caffeine helps mobilize fat as an energy source.

Another optimal time to perform your aerobic activity is late afternoon, when your metabolism begins to slow down. Try to do it as close to 5:00 P.M. as possible and always before dinner. (For this same reason, late-night dinners are problematic. Most of the food you ingest then won't be converted into fuel. Instead, while you're sleeping, your body will turn it into fat and store it in all the wrong places.)

If you do your aerobic activity prior to eating a sensible dinner, you'll boost your metabolism for up to 3 hours and burn far more calories that way. (For a complete discussion of the Action Hero nutrition plan, see chapter 4.)

You can do aerobic activities 4 to 6 days a week, even twice a day or after your weight-lifting workout and cardio test. In this case, though, work on your abs after your aerobic session.

And remember: *Don't overdo it.* Take at least 1 day off each week. That way, you can refresh yourself for the next week's workouts.

STAGE TWO

You'll notice that the following workouts are much more intense and challenging than those offered in Stage One. You'll also add an extra day of weight lifting to the week. During Stage Two, you might feel fatigued, thirsty, or even depleted sometimes. But overall you'll feel stronger, more athletic, and energized, and you'll enjoy a sense of well-being. So accept the challenges that this level gives; you'll always come out a winner in the end.

Increasing the intensity of your workout allows you to improve on four different levels: strength, endurance, stamina, and balance. You'll use the same exercises as in Stage One, but you'll increase the weight according to your individual improvements. Continue gauging your weight loads based on the percentage guidelines discussed earlier. In this way, you can create an individual training schedule that's the optimum for you.

As an example, here's a weekly program designed for the average 33-year-old man who works 8 hours a day, 5 days per week, and wants to lose 20 pounds.

Sunday: Aerobic activity for 20 to 60 minutes

Monday: Day One workout and 20 minutes of aerobic activity

Tuesday: Aerobic activity for 20 to 60 minutes

Wednesday: Day Two workout and 20 minutes of aerobic activity

Thursday: Aerobic activity for 20 to 60 minutes

Friday: Day Three workout and 20 minutes of aerobic activity

Saturday: Rest

For those of you who don't want to lose any weight but just want to get stronger and healthier, here's a weekly program for you.

Sunday: Rest

Monday: Day One workout

Tuesday: Aerobic activity for 20 to 60 minutes

Wednesday: Day Two workout

Thursday: Rest

Friday: Day Three workout

Saturday: Rest

Day One

Here are the specific exercises to perform on Day One workout days. (*Note:* Detailed descriptions of all these exercises appear in the "Body Sculpting" section, which begins on page 110.) Start with a 10-minute warmup and mild stretching for 1 minute, then go straight into the weight lifting.

DAY ONE (FIRST PART)	SETS	REPS	PERCENTAGES
Pulldown	4	12	50-65-80-80
Superset w/			
Vertical Bench Press Machine	4	12	50-65-80-80
Superset w/			
E-Z Barbell Curl	4	12	50-65-80-80
Superset w/			
Triceps Pushdown	4	12	50-65-80-80

After the first part of the workout, you'll increase the repetitions from 12 to 15 for the second part. You'll also need to decrease the amount of weight you lift in order to accommodate the extra 3 reps. This doesn't mean, though, that you'll change the intensity of your workout. That should remain at 80 percent.

As you'll soon discover, you can easily change the intensity of the workout simply by adding or stripping off the weight, or by increasing or decreasing the reps. Depending on how quickly your cardiovascular condition improves, you can also decrease the amount of time you rest between sets.

DAY ONE (SECOND PART)	SETS	REPS	PERCENTAGE
Vertical Pull Machine	2	15	80
Superset w/			
Cable-Cross Machine	2	15	80
Superset w/			
Speedy Alternating Dumbbells	2	15	80
Superset w/			
Dippy	2	15	80

After you complete these sets, you'll really notice fatigue in your muscles. Follow the workout with a mild cardio test as described in Stage One, but increase the level of intensity on the machine (to level 10 or higher) for a longer period of time.

Here's an example.

2 minutes—level 9 at 90 rpm

11 minutes—level 10 at 90 rpm

1 minute—level 8 at 75 rpm

Finally, finish up with the abdominal muscles, but take no breaks during the reps and no longer than 20 to 30 seconds between the sets. If you still have energy after one round of these exercises, then repeat the round.

Crunch—30 to 40 reps

Side-to-Side—20 reps on each side

Knee Lift—20 reps

Rocky's—30 to 50 reps on each side

Day Two

Here's something completely new to add to the equation. After your warmup, drink a little water and get ready to train the toughest muscle group in your body—your legs. The best exercises to train the legs require total involvement of the whole body. Rest minimally between exercises, if you can.

DAY TWO	SETS	REPS	PERCENTAGES
Leg Press	4	12	50-60-70-70
Superset w/			
Leg Curl (preferably seated)	4	12	50-60-70-70
Cross-Step Lunge	2	12	steps each side

No supersets here. Just alternate from one leg to the other. Take a short break after each 12 reps, if you need to. When you're done, move on to the next exercise.

Leg extension	2	15	70

Same here, no supersets. Do one set of Leg Extensions, take a 1- to 2-minute break, then do another.

No cardio test on Day Two. It's more like a ride in the park: 10 minutes on level 8 at 90 rpm. The purpose of this is to flush from the leg muscles all the lactic acid and toxic buildup. It significantly reduces leg soreness that you might experience the day after your leg workout.

If it seems, for some reason, that the 70 percent sets are too easy after the first workout, jack up the weight the next time around so you'll be training at 80 percent of your capacity. Don't get carried away, though. You have to get stronger first. No harm is done if you take it too easy in your first workout.

Day Three

You're back to working the upper body, shoulders, and arms. Because biceps and triceps are the smallest major muscle groups in the body, you can train them more frequently. They can't be trained as hard as the bigger muscle groups such as the legs, back, and chest. However, they need less time to recover.

DAY THREE	SETS	REPS	PERCENTAGES
Shoulder Press Machine	4	12	50-65-80-80
Superset w/			
Straight Barbell Curl	3	15	70
Upright Dumbbell Row	2	12	80
Superset w/			
Overhead Rope Extension	3	15	70
Side Laterals (with dumbbells)	2	15	80

Same as with the Leg Extension on Day Two. Do the Side Laterals (with dumbbells) by themselves; no supersets. Do one set of 15 reps, take a 1- to 2-minute break, then do another set.

We're done with the lifting, which leaves us with a mild cardio test and abdominals. Use the same principles as described in the Stage Two, Day One workout.

STAGE THREE

Most of you should be ready to enter Stage Three after spending 4 weeks in Stage One and another 4 to 6 weeks in Stage Two. This is for the serious athlete who's ready to reach new heights in his Action Hero training program.

I've designed Stage Three in a way that allows you to design your own AH workout routine. Pick your own intensity level, frequency, and favorite exercises. This will be the last exercise book you'll ever need to buy. Even those of you who have already reached a high level of muscle development will get stronger, more muscular, and leaner.

Let's start with what you can expect from Stage Three.

• Do a high-intensity 7-minute warmup and 1 minute of mild stretching before the weight-lifting routine and a 15-minute cardio test after the routine. You can expect to sweat bullets after you're done with this routine. But you'll also be ready to take on the workload of the Stage Three Action Hero workouts. Then you'll continue with the abdominal workout from Stage Two, but with the ability to construct your own personalized abdominal routine.

• You'll become acquainted with the all-important 85-to-95-percent-of-your-capacity set, or HIS (high-intensity set). After your first warmup set at 50 percent capacity, and after your second warmup set at 70 percent capacity, you'll really blast your muscles with a couple of sets at 85 to 95 percent capacity. It's all about intensity.

• You'll become more familiar with the exercises and learn more about how to choose basic, concentration, or isolation exercises according to your own personalized workout pattern.

• You'll encounter more cycles during this stage of the program, but without compromising the effectiveness of the AH
training system.

• Once you've chosen a cycle that fits into your time schedule
and works with your other commitments, you'll have to stick to
it for at least 3 months before you notice any substantial
changes to your body. No worries; it won't be boring, because
you can change the exercises from workout to workout—as
long as you keep the same cycle and the same sequence of body
parts with their exercises (more about this later when I talk
about building your own AH workout).

I prefer to train every other day. This allows me to train all the
major muscle groups roughly twice in an 8- to 9-day period, depending
on the actual size and training intensity of the muscle group. I don't
hold to a weekly pattern. I don't believe the body functions this way. I
train whenever I can and whenever my body allows it.

Even though I usually don't stray from the every-other-day cycle,
there are days when I can't train. What do I do when I skip a day? The
next day, I'll train the muscle groups that I was supposed to train, and
the very next day after that I train again, in accordance with my cycle.
Even though it's 2 days in a row, I feel it's okay because I had an extra
day off. After that, I resume my regular cycle of 1 day on, 1 day off.

I have a few clients who don't like to train more than 3 days per week
and prefer to take the weekends off. For those of you who feel the same
way, I've come up with a three-workouts-per-week cycle. It's a great way
to work out, and it gives you enough time to think about things other
than your body.

Before we begin, though, let's review some basic terminology that
you may have forgotten from previous sections of this book.

When we talk about your warmup set being executed at 50 percent
of your capacity, the weight that you use should be light enough so that
you don't fatigue the muscles. A good barometer: If you can comfortably

execute 12 reps on a particular exercise, this is the weight you should start with. When we talk about your second warmup set being executed at 70 percent of your capacity, however, you want to use a weight that you can do with strict form and without any real strain. Your muscles should experience a tingling sensation and a slight sense of fatigue.

Finally, the weight to use on your HIS should be heavy enough so that the last few reps are done with extreme effort, without compromising form.

Before you begin, allow me to set the ground rules for building your own AH workout.

- Ask yourself which cycle suits you best, depending on which days you want to train.

- Start building your AH workout by picking two exercises to start your first superset.

- Pick two new exercises for your next superset, according to the instructions given in your particular cycle of choice.

- Work all the muscle groups with the appropriate exercises.

- Go to the gym with your self-made AH workout and start with your first warmup set, then your second warmup set, and finally your HIS sets. Once you get into the groove, you'll think it's the easiest workout in the world.

This program should keep you occupied for several months or more. However, you can keep changing the workouts by choosing different exercises. And, of course, as you get stronger you can up the weight of each exercise. Just never compromise the form and never decrease the amount of reps below 8 on your basic exercises. Keep the reps constant (12 to 15) on all the concentration and isolation exercises.

Note the 75 to 95 percentage set in this stage. It means you pick a weight that feels nice and comfortable on the first set, but because of the multiple sets, the fatigue factor will kick in and soon enough you'll experience an 85 to 95 percent effect on your muscles.

Option A/Variation 1
Every-other-day, full-body cycle (8 days)

Day One: chest, light biceps, light side deltoids, and triceps

Day Two: back, light triceps, light rear deltoids, and biceps

Day Three: shoulders, light biceps, and triceps

Day Four: legs

DAY ONE	SETS	REPS	PERCENTAGES
Incline Dumbbell Press	4	12	50-70-HIS-HIS
Or any other B chest exercise			
Superset w/			
E-Z Barbell Curl	4	15	75 to 95
Or any other B, C, or I biceps exercise			
Vertical Bench Press Machine	2	12	HIS-HIS
Or any other B or C chest exercise			
Superset w/			
E-Z Barbell Curl	1	15	75 to 95
Side Laterals (with dumbbells)	3	15	75 to 95
Or any other I shoulder exercise			
Superset w/			
French Press	3	10	70-HIS-HIS
Or any other B triceps exercise			
Pec Deck or Butterfly Machine	2	15	HIS-HIS
Or any other I chest exercise			
Superset w/			
French Press	2	10	HIS-HIS

Basic (B)   Concentration (C)   Isolation (I)

DAY TWO	SETS	REPS	PERCENTAGES
Low-Pulley Row	4	12	50-70-HIS-HIS
Or any other B back exercise			
Superset w/			
Overhead Rope Extension	4	15	75 to 95
Or any other B, C, or I triceps exercise			
Lat Pulldown (wide grip)	2	12	HIS-HIS
Or any other B or C back exercise			
Superset w/			
Overhead Rope Extension	1	15	75 to 95
Rear Deltoids with Cables	3	15	75 to 95
Or any other rear deltoids variation			
Superset w/			
Alternating Dumbbell Curl	3	10	70-HIS-HIS
Or any other B biceps exercise			
Lat Flex	2	15	HIS-HIS
Superset w/			
Alternating Dumbbell Curl	2	10	HIS-HIS

DAY THREE	SETS	REPS	PERCENTAGES
Standing Dumbbell Press	4	12	50-70-HIS-HIS
Or any other B shoulder exercise			
Superset w/			
Speedy Alternating Dumbbells	3	15	75 to 95
Or any other B, C, or I biceps exercise			
Dippy	3	15	body weight
Or any other B, C, or I triceps exercise			
Superset w/			
Upright Dumbbell Row	2	12	HIS-HIS
Or any of the other variations of upright rows			
Side Laterals (with cables)—double	2	15	HIS-HIS
Do two sets back to back with a 1-minute rest between sets.			

(continued)

DAY THREE (CONT.)	SETS	REPS	PERCENTAGES
Front Laterals (with cables)—double	2	15	HIS-HIS

Do two sets back to back with a 1-minute rest between sets.

DAY FOUR	SETS	REPS	PERCENTAGES
Leg Press	5	12	50-70-HIS-HIS-HIS

Or Squat

Superset w/

	SETS	REPS	PERCENTAGES
Seated Leg Curl	5	12	50-70-HIS-HIS-HIS

Or any other hamstrings exercise.
The third HIS set in both exercises is optional.

	SETS	REPS	PERCENTAGES
Lunge on Smith Machine	3	12	70-HIS-HIS

Or any C exercise for quads/glutes

	SETS	REPS	PERCENTAGES
Leg Extension	2	15	HIS-HIS

Superset w/

	SETS	REPS	PERCENTAGES
Butt Squeeze	2	15	body weight

There is no cardio test on Day Four, only a 5-minute cooldown on the bike (level 8 at 75 rpm).

Option A/Variation 2
Every-other-day, full-body cycle (8 days)

Day One: chest, biceps, light side deltoids, and light triceps

Day Two: back, triceps, light rear deltoids, and light biceps

Day Three: shoulders, light biceps, and triceps

Day Four: legs

DAY ONE	SETS	REPS	PERCENTAGES
Incline Dumbbell Press	4	12	50-70-HIS-HIS

Superset w/

	SETS	REPS	PERCENTAGES
Biceps exercise chosen from B exercises	4	10	50-70-HIS-HIS

DAY ONE (CONT.)	SETS	REPS	PERCENTAGES
Vertical Bench Press Machine	2	12	HIS-HIS
Superset w/			
Biceps exercise chosen from C or I	2	15	HIS-HIS
Side Laterals (with dumbbells)	3	15	75 to 95
Superset w/			
Triceps exercises chosen from B or C	3	15	75 to 95
Pec Deck or Butterfly Machine	2	15	HIS-HIS
Superset w/			
Same triceps exercise as in previous superset	2	15	75 to 95

DAY TWO	SETS	REPS	PERCENTAGES
Low-Pulley Row	4	12	50-70-HIS-HIS
Superset w/			
Triceps exercise chosen from B exercises	4	10	50-70-HIS-HIS
Lat Pulldown (wide grip)	4	12	HIS-HIS
Superset w/			
Triceps exercise chosen from C	2	15	HIS-HIS
Rear Deltoids with Cables	3	15	75 to 95
Superset w/			
Biceps exercise chosen from B, C, or I	3	15	75 to 95
Lat Flex	2	15	HIS-HIS
Superset w/			
Same biceps exercise as in previous superset	2	15	75-95

DAY THREE	SETS	REPS	PERCENTAGES
Standing Dumbbell Press	4	12	50-70-HIS-HIS
Or any other B shoulder exercise			
Superset w/			
Speedy Alternating Dumbbells	3	15	75 to 95
Or any other B, C, or I biceps exercise			

Basic (B)   Concentration (C)   Isolation (I)

(continued)

DAY THREE (CONT.)	SETS	REPS	PERCENTAGES
Dippy	3	15	body weight
Or any other B, C, or I triceps exercise			
Superset w/			
Upright Dumbbell Row	2	12	HIS-HIS
Or any of the other variations of upright row			
Side Laterals (with cables)—double	2	15	HIS-HIS
Do two sets back to back with a 1-minute rest between sets.			
Front Laterals (with cables)—double	2	15	HIS-HIS
Do two sets back to back with a 1-minute rest between sets.			

DAY FOUR	SETS	REPS	PERCENTAGES
Leg Press	5	12	50-70-HIS-HIS-HIS
Or Squat			
Superset w/			
Seated Leg Curl	5	12	50-70-HIS-HIS-HIS
Or any other hamstrings exercise. The third HIS set in both exercises is optional.			
Lunge on Smith Machine	3	12	70-HIS-HIS
Or any C exercise for quads/glutes			
Leg Extension	2	15	HIS-HIS
Superset w/			
Butt Squeeze	2	15	body weight

There is no cardio test on Day Four, only a 5-minute cooldown on the bike (level 8 at 75 rpm).

This next cycle is for those who need to stick to a 7-day pattern. It's probably one of the hardest cycles, but again, because of the adequate rest time between workouts (Wednesday, Saturday, and Sunday), it's still a great way to get in the best possible condition of your life. If, for some reason, this cycle is too strenuous, you can always use option C.

Option B
2 days on, 1 day off, 2 days on, 2 days off (7 days)

Monday: back, light triceps, light rear deltoids, and biceps

Tuesday: chest, light biceps, light side deltoids, and triceps

Thursday: legs

Friday: shoulders, light biceps, and triceps

MONDAY	SETS	REPS	PERCENTAGES
Low-Pulley Row	4	12	50-70-HIS-HIS
Or any other B back exercise			
Superset w/			
Overhead Rope Extension	4	15	75 to 95
Or any other B, C, or I triceps exercise			
Lat Pulldown (wide grip)	2	12	HIS-HIS
Or any other B or C back exercise			
Superset w/			
Overhead Rope Extension	1	15	75 to 95
Rear Deltoids with Cables	3	15	75 to 95
Or any other rear deltoids variation			
Superset w/			
Alternating Dumbbell Curl	3	10	70-HIS-HIS
Or any other B biceps exercise			
Lat Flex	2	15	HIS-HIS
Superset w/			
Alternating Dumbbell Curl	2	10	HIS-HIS

TUESDAY	SETS	REPS	PERCENTAGES
Incline Dumbbell Press	4	12	50-70-HIS-HIS
Or any other B chest exercise			
Superset w/			
E-Z Barbell Curl	4	15	75 to 95
Or any other B, C, or I biceps exercise			

(continued)

TUESDAY (CONT.)	SETS	REPS	PERCENTAGES
Vertical Bench Press Machine	2	12	HIS-HIS
Or any other B or C chest exercise			
Superset w/			
E-Z Barbell Curl	1	15	75 to 95
Side Laterals (with dumbbells)	3	15	75 to 95
Or any other I shoulder exercise			
Superset w/			
French Press	3	10	70-HIS-HIS
Or any other B triceps exercise			
Pec Deck or Butterfly Machine	2	15	HIS-HIS
Or any other I chest exercise			
Superset w/			
French Press	2	10	HIS-HIS

THURSDAY	SETS	REPS	PERCENTAGES
Leg Press	5	12	50-70-HIS-HIS-HIS
Or Squat			
Superset w/			
Seated Leg Curl	5	12	50-70-HIS-HIS-HIS
Or any other hamstrings exercise.			
The third HIS set in both exercises is optional.			
Lunge on Smith Machine	3	12	70-HIS-HIS
Or any C exercise for quads/glutes			
Leg Extension	2	15	HIS-HIS
Superset w/			
Butt Squeeze	2	15	body weight

Basic (B)   Concentration (C)   Isolation (I)

There is no cardio test on Thursday, only a 5-minute cooldown on the bike (level 8 at 75 rpm).

FRIDAY	SETS	REPS	PERCENTAGES
Standing Dumbbell Press	4	12	50-70-HIS-HIS
Or any other B shoulder exercise			
Superset w/			
Speedy Alternating Dumbbells	3	15	75 to 95
Or any other B, C, or I biceps exercise			
Dippy	3	15	body weight
Or any other B, C, or I triceps exercise			
Superset w/			
Upright Dumbbell Row	2	12	HIS-HIS
Or any of the other variations of upright row			
Side Laterals (with cables)—double	2	15	HIS-HIS
Do two sets back to back with a 1-minute rest between sets.			
Front Laterals (with cables)—double	2	15	HIS-HIS
Do two sets back to back with a 1-minute rest between sets.			

Option C
3-days-a-week cycle (7 days)

Monday: back, chest, light shoulders, and light arms

Wednesday: legs

Friday: shoulders and arms

MONDAY	SETS	REPS	PERCENTAGES
Low-Pulley Row	4	12	50-70-HIS-HIS
Or any other B back exercise			
Superset w/			
Incline Smith Machine Press	4	12	50-70-HIS-HIS
Or any other B chest exercise			

Basic (B) Concentration (C) Isolation (I)

(continued)

MONDAY (CONT.)	SETS	REPS	PERCENTAGES
Superset w/			
Side Laterals (with dumbbells)—double	4	15	75 to 95
Gravetron-Supported Chinup	2	12	HIS-HIS
Or any other C back exercise			
Superset w/			
Flat Smith Machine Press	2	12	HIS-HIS
Or any other C chest exercise			
Superset w/			
Side Laterals (with dumbbells)—double	1	15	75 to 95
Cable-Cross Pulldown	2	15	HIS-HIS
Or any other I back exercise			
Superset w/			
Pec Deck or Butterfly Machine	2	15	HIS-HIS
Or any other I chest exercise			
Speedy Alternating Dumbbells	3	15	75 to 95
Or any other biceps exercise			
Superset w/			
Dippy	3	15	75 to 95
Or any other triceps exercise			

WEDNESDAY	SETS	REPS	PERCENTAGES
Leg Press	5	12	50-70-HIS-HIS-HIS
Superset w/			
Leg Extension	5	15	75 to 95
Superset w/			
Lying Leg Curl	5	12	50-70-HIS-HIS-HIS

After each round, take about a 2-minute break. As you get more conditioned, you can make the breaks between your sets shorter.

Basic (B)   Concentration (C)   Isolation (I)

WEDNESDAY (CONT.)	SETS	REPS	PERCENTAGES
One-Legged Skater Lunge	2–3	12–15	body weight

Or any other lunge-type exercise.
Take a 1- to 2-minute break after finishing all reps of each set.

	SETS	REPS	PERCENTAGES
Butt Squeeze	2–3	15	body weight

As you get in better condition, try holding a 10-pound plate in front of your chest
(cross your arms to hold it). Take about a 1-minute break after each set.

FRIDAY	SETS	REPS	PERCENTAGES
Seated Dumbbell Press	4	12	50-70-HIS-HIS

Or any other B shoulder exercise

Superset w/

	SETS	REPS	PERCENTAGES
E-Z Barbell Curl	4	10	50-70-HIS-HIS

Or any other B biceps exercise

	SETS	REPS	PERCENTAGES
Upright Dumbbell Row	2	12	HIS-HIS

Or any other C shoulder exercise

Superset w/

	SETS	REPS	PERCENTAGES
E-Z Barbell Curl	2	10	HIS-HIS
French Press	2	10	50-70

Superset w/

	SETS	REPS	PERCENTAGES
Front Laterals (with dumbbells)	2	15	HIS-HIS

Or any other I shoulder exercise

	SETS	REPS	PERCENTAGES
French Press	2	10	HIS-HIS

Or any other B triceps exercise

Superset w/

	SETS	REPS	PERCENTAGES
Front Laterals (with dumbbells)	2	15	HIS-HIS

Or any other I shoulder exercise

	SETS	REPS	PERCENTAGES
French Press	2	10	HIS-HIS

No supersets here, just take a 1- to 2-minute break between the last 2 sets.

Circuit Training: A Giant Step Forward

Here's a circuit-training workout, a multiple superset of exercises. This program is executed over a 3-day cycle with a minimum of 2 to 3 days between workouts. Move at your own pace. It's great if you're just coming back to the gym after a layoff or if you just want a breather from heavy lifting. I almost always stick to my every-other-day regimen (Option A, Variation 2). But occasionally, I alternate with this program.

Start with a warmup on a bike or some other cardio machine. Remember to step it up and make it challenging. Follow with a giant set of more than two exercises. If you need to take a short 30-second break between sets, go ahead. At the end of the round—which includes all five exercises—take a 1- to 2-minute break.

DAY ONE	SETS	REPS	PERCENTAGE
Lat Pulldown (medium grip)	2	15	70 to 95
Superset w/			
Incline Smith Machine Press	2	15	70 to 95
Superset w/			
Upright Dumbbell Row	2	15	70 to 95
Superset w/			
E-Z Barbell Curl	2	15	70 to 95
Superset w/			
Triceps Pushdown	2	15	70 to 95
Finished? Move on to the next giant set, executed in the same way as the previous giant set.			
Vertical Pull Machine (lower or upper grip)	2	15	70 to 95
Superset w/			
Vertical Bench Press Machine	2	15	70 to 95
Superset w/			
Side Laterals (with dumbbells)	2	15	70 to 95
Superset w/			
Speedy Alternating Dumbbells	2	15	70 to 95
Superset w/			
Dippy	2	15	70 to 95

Follow the Day One workout with either a 15-minute cardio test on the bike or pushing The Cart. Or you can go right into an aerobic session on the treadmill for 20 to 40 minutes. Make sure you keep your heartbeat in the 120 to 130 beats-per-minute range. Never run, always walk, and after you increase the treadmill's incline, watch that your lower back doesn't strain. When you're at the end of this session, cool down by riding your bike at level 7 and pedaling at a speed of 75 rpm, or walk slowly on the treadmill for 2 minutes.

DAY TWO	SETS	REPS	PERCENTAGE
Leg Press	3	15	70 to 95
Superset w/			
Seated Leg Curl	3	15	70 to 95
Cross-Step Lunge	3	15	85 to 95

Do 12 to 15 lunges on each leg, take a break for 1 to 2 minutes, and do it again for a total of three times. As you improve, consider holding dumbbells in your hands. However, never compromise form.

	SETS	REPS	PERCENTAGE
Lying Leg Curl	2	15	70 to 95
Superset w/			
Leg Extension	2	15	70 to 95

End with a 5-minute, low-intensity cooldown on a stationary bike. Keep it at level 8 and 75 rpm.

DAY THREE	SETS	REPS	PERCENTAGE
Vertical Pull Machine	4	15	70 to 95
(lower or upper grip)			
Superset w/			
Vertical Bench Press Machine	4	15	70 to 95
Superset w/			
Side Laterals	4	15	70 to 95
Superset w/			
Seated Dumbbell Press	4	15	70 to 95
Superset w/			
Overhead Rope Extension	4	15	70 to 95

All five sets are executed in succession with only a 1-minute break after completion of each giant set; you're doing four. It's a killer workout, but you'll feel pumped afterwards and have energy to spare. After this workout, do a 15-minute cardio test or an aerobic session as described in Day One.

THE ZIG-ZAG EFFECT

This is a good place to stop for a moment and consider what I like to call the Zig-Zag Effect. Typically, during the beginning of a workout, your body's full of energy and your muscles are loaded with glucogen (muscle energy). You're ready to go at it full blast. After the first few warmup sets, you add just enough resistance weight to reach that all-important HIS, or roughly 85 to 95 percent of your personal capacity. With a 1- to 2-minute break after your first HIS, your body recovers for a strong second HIS.

This is about when the first signs of muscle fatigue start to surface. The first "good" damage has been done; you've broken down the muscle tissue and given it permission to recover, grow, and develop bigger and stronger than before.

When you work out at full capacity for set after set, you establish a cumulative fatigue rate. With every set you complete, you become a little more tired. Even with 1- to 2-minute breaks between sets, you don't recover as well as you did after the previous set. You just continue to add to the muscle fatigue. The third HIS becomes even harder, the fourth HIS even harder than that, until you've exhausted the muscle completely.

No worries. This is exactly how it's supposed to work.

However, too many HISs in a row can cause the body to break down muscle tissue faster than your body can rebuild it during the recovery periods. To avoid this common pitfall, you must work out at a rate that your body can handle in terms of recovery.

Again, no worries. My system will never allow you to get there. With my system, you'll train harder and more efficiently than you've ever trained before. What's not to like?

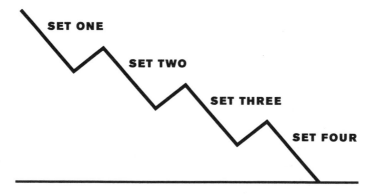

The downward line represents you doing a set of 8, 10, 12, or even 15 reps. The upward line represents the muscle trained and your rest between sets. Remember, even though you take a break between sets, you'll never match the energy you had at the beginning of Set One. Your muscles become progressively more fatigued . . . until you've reached that all-important horizontal line.

As a rule, never cross the horizontal line, or what I like to call the danger zone. In the illustration on the opposite page, you can see that at the end of Set Three, you're still above the danger zone—safe and with a successfully completed workout. By the time your next workout comes around, you'll train even harder and heavier than the workout before.

It's the accumulation of training too hard, too long, and too often that will take you over the top and will do you more harm than good. So much harm, in fact, that you'll end up drifting away from your ultimate goal of becoming an Action Hero.

Rule of thumb: Hit each muscle as hard as you can, but never too much. Stay out of the danger zone.

ACTION HERO PROGRESS DIAGRAM

In your time of rest between your AH workouts, you should start to feel stronger, more energetic, and more confident. This sense of well-being should continue, and that's what I call Zig-Zag Upward and Onward.

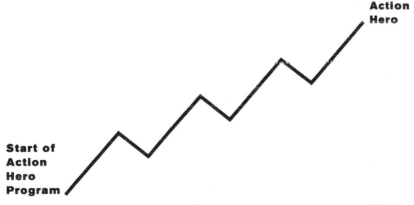

Every peak indicates you at the beginning of your AH workout. Every valley indicates you at the end of your AH workout and at the beginning of your recuperation period. As you can see, you'll build more muscle than you've broken down. Every peak is a little bit higher than the previous one.

You enable this by giving your body adequate amounts of rest and building blocks—such as good, healthy nutrition and supplementation—in your time of recuperation between workouts.

The sky's the limit. Remember: "There's never best, but always better!"

Jørgy's Workout Cycle

Since I have an erratic work schedule and a busy family life, I rely on the every-other-day workout cycle. Some weeks, I admit, I work out 2 days in a row, then go back to the every-other-day approach. But for the most part, I'm fairly consistent.

Here's the breakdown of my personal Action Hero workout cycle. I do my warmup or light set at 50 percent of capacity, my second set at 70 percent of capacity, and my cruise weight or HIS between 85 and 95 percent of capacity. (A light set means I'll do 15 reps. I'll pick a weight that's not easy but doable, which will pre-exhaust the other muscle groups.) Use my cycle, if you want, to construct your own workout.

I start with a 7-minute cardio workout on the bike. For the record, my legs have always been my strongest muscle group. It's easy for me to get them strong, big, and defined. Nevertheless, I always train them as hard as I can. Not so much because I need the strenuous workout, but because I get stronger in all the other muscle groups, as well—back, chest, shoulders, and arms. I have all my clients train their legs as hard as they can. It also helps increase your metabolic rate.

DAY ONE	SETS	REPS	WEIGHT
Incline Smith Machine Press	4	12	25-50-75-75 lb on each side
Superset w/			
E-Z Barbell Curl	4	10	10-20-30-30 lb on each side
Flat Smith Machine Press	2	12	70-70 lb on each side
Superset w/			
E-Z Barbell Curl	2	10	30-30 lb on each side

For biceps, the same as the previous superset.

DAY ONE (CONT.)	SETS	REPS	WEIGHT
Side Laterals (with cables)—double	3	15	40-40-40 lb
Superset w/			
Triceps Pushdown (narrow grip)	3	15	120-120-120 lb
Pec Deck or Butterfly Machine	2	15	70-70 lb
Superset w/			
Triceps Pushdown (narrow grip)	2	15	120-120 lb

Since I'm already at my Action Hero weight goal of 200 pounds, I don't always do a postworkout cardio test. For health reasons and to stay at peak condition, I'll do it only one or two times a week. But then, I also play ice hockey and basketball with my son a couple of times a week, and I walk to work almost every day.

DAY TWO	SETS	REPS	WEIGHT
Lying T-Bar Machine	4	12	45-70-95-95 lb
Superset w/			
French Press (E-Z bar)	4	10	10-20-30-30 lb on each side
Pulldown (medium grip)	2	12	120-120 lb
Superset w/			
French Press (E-Z bar)	2	10	30-30 lb on each side
Rear Deltoids with Cables	3	15	20-20-20 lb
Superset w/			
Straight Barbell Curl (wide grip)	3	15	10-10-10 lb on each side
Lat Flex	2	15	90-90 lb
Superset w/			
Straight Barbell Curl (wide grip)	2	15	10-10 lb on each side

I finish Day Two with a cardio test.

ACTION!

Action Hero: Robert Towne

Career accomplishments: Director and screenwriter. Well-known for his screenplays *Chinatown* and *Mission Impossible.* Robert also wrote the screenplays for *The Last Detail* and *Shampoo,* which were both nominated for Oscars for Best Original Screenplay. Among others, he wrote and directed *Tequila Sunrise* and *Personal Best.*

Physical goals: After being on "nonactive duty," Robert wanted to regenerate his body. We focused on weight loss, increased muscle tone, and improved cardiovascular condition.

Training program: A 35-minute superset and giant set workout routines, followed by 45 minutes of aerobic activity. Later that day he'd do another aerobic activity, either walking on the treadmill or hiking up a steep hill in his neighborhood. Or he'd swim laps in the 25-yard pool in his backyard.

Results: Strong as an ox, with the respiratory system of a 27-year-old (these are his doctor's words). He was able to swim fast for 45 minutes straight with a heart rate of about 170 beats per minute.

Even though Robert is not *that* young, he could fool you with the intensity of his workouts. I've never encountered anyone like him. You'd think he really was 27 years old, given the weights he's pushing in the gym. Not only that, he'll swim 2,500 yards any day of the week in record time.

When Robert and I started working together, he was about 30 pounds overweight and very, very sedentary, so we had to start up slowly. During the first 2 weeks, we worked out just every other day, but soon we were up to 6 days a week and twice a day for most of those days. Robert told me once that he thought the advantage of having a trainer is that you don't have to think about anything: You just do what you're told.

After about 9 weeks, Robert was in tip-top condition and had lost 32 pounds and gained 10 pounds of muscle (thus, he lost a total of about 42 pounds of fat).

Intensifying your workout load and increasing the frequency *and* duration of each aerobic activity will help increase your muscle tone, your cardiovascular condition, and your basal metabolic rate to burn more body fat.

DAY THREE	SETS	REPS	WEIGHT
Seated Dumbbell Press	4	12	25-40-55-55 lb
Superset w/			
Upright Dumbbell Row	4	12	20-25-25-25 lb
Superset w/			
Speedy Alternating Dumbbells	4	15	25-25-25-25 lb
Seated Bent-Over Laterals with Dumbbells	3	12	20-20-20 lb
Superset w/			
Overhead Rope Extension	3	15	70-70-70 lb
Front Laterals (with cables)	2	15	40-40 lb
Superset w/			
Overhead Rope Extension	2	15	70-70 lb

DAY FOUR	SETS	REPS	WEIGHT
Leg Press	5	2-12-8-8-15	200-400-800-800-600 lb
Superset w/			
Stiff-Legged Deadlift (with dumbbells)	5	12	30-40-50-50-50 lb

These weights are not my max, but they work my legs sufficiently to have muscle-building effects at the end of my routine.

Any kind of lunge	3	10–20	

Sometimes I do heavy Lunges on Smith Machine (10 reps per leg). Other times I do Cross-Step Lunges (as many as 20 steps per leg). Also, I take breaks based on my heartbeat—never under 100 beats per minute or when I'm not out of breath anymore after finishing a set.

Leg Extension	2–3	15	100 lb
Superset w/			
Lying Leg Curl	2–3	15	70 lb

I always do my 5 minutes on the bike right after—low intensity and low rpm.

8

THE
FLEXIBILITY
FACTOR

OST FITNESS PROFESSIONALS claim that their clients must stay flexible to reach their peak physical potential, and I agree. In my Action Hero workouts, I stress the importance of using the various joints' and muscles' full range of motion in all workouts, and more specifically, in all exercises.

Sometimes a joint is restricted in its normal range of motion by genetic disposition, the joint structure itself, connective tissue elasticity within the muscles, tendons, and even neuromuscular coordination. One way to stay flexible is to focus on the way you stretch, which will help you balance muscle groups that might be overused during physical training sessions.

There are two basic types of flexibility: static and dynamic. Every body should possess at least a minimum level of static flexibility, the kind of stretching that involves a slow, gradual, and controlled elongation of the muscle through a full range of its motion. For example, when stretching the calf muscle, you should always lean over the forward knee until you feel a pull, without pain, and hold this position for about 15 seconds. This is a low-intensity, long-duration technique that causes very little trauma to the muscle. A big advantage of static flexibility is that it helps you do your AH workouts without any restrictions. Joints will move about freely, and muscles will respond more readily because of the improved bloodflow. Static flexibility will give you a better pump, along with the energy to build muscle tissue and joints more rapidly.

But stretching shouldn't take precedence over the warmup and strength-conditioning portions of your Action Hero training program. Too much stretching, in my opinion, can hamper the strength of your joints and ligaments. Your joints should be relatively stiff for your work-

INJURIES

Even when you have a slight muscle pull from training—maybe because you lost your focus for a minute, or you simply trained a little too hard—you don't have to freak out and quit. Lighter workouts can actually speed up the healing process.

Here's why.

When at rest, muscles get stiff and have a tendency to atrophy roughly 72 hours after your last workout. Your muscles are actually weaker and therefore the strain on the injured muscle is greater. In order to avoid muscle atrophy, continue training to flush the blood and all its waste products out of the injured muscle and revive it with freshly oxygenated blood and other nutrients. This will shorten the recovery time.

However, don't think that the injury is completely healed. It's not, though it's on the mend. Keep working out and keep increasing the intensity in accordance with how the injured muscle feels the day after each workout.

outs. Warm them up, certainly, but don't stretch them out. There's a difference.

Why You Must Stretch

A full range of motion in all your muscle groups means you'll get the most out of your workouts. Here are some of the specific benefits you can expect when you include stretching in your routine.

Increased physical efficiency and performance. A flexible joint has the ability to move farther in its range and requires less energy to do so.

Decreased risk of injury. Even though there's no scientific proof to back this up, in my experience it's clear that flexible muscles and joints are less likely to be strained by overuse or a sudden, incorrect movement. More flexibility, in combination with a warmup on the bike and your AH warmup sets, should guarantee an almost injury-free workout.

Increased blood supply and nutrients to the joints. During flexibility training, tissue temperature increases, which in turn improves circulation, nutrient transport, and elasticity in and around the joints.

Increased quality and quantity of joint fluid. Stretching slows down joint-degenerative processes.

Increased neuromuscular coordination. Overall coordination in your workout, such as executing the exercises correctly, will increase with improved flexibility. Studies have shown that nerve impulses shooting from the brain and back again travel at a faster rate than when the body hasn't been stretched.

Reduced muscular soreness and stiffness. I don't believe in a long, intense stretch session before an AH workout. However, I do believe in short, mild stretching right before, during, and after workouts, and between high-intensity exercises. This helps stimulate the blood to flow in those stagnant muscles and joints. You'll feel more limber and relaxed after this kind of stretching session and also the next day.

Improved muscular balance and posture. To correct a slouching posture, you must stretch your pectoral muscles and strengthen the muscles in your back. This will open up your chest and straighten your back. Another good trick to instantly improve your posture is to take a deep breath and hold it for a second. Notice how your chest rises and your spine straightens. Now, hold this position and breathe out slowly. Imagine lifting your heart to the sky.

Decreased risk of lower-back pain. Stretching and strengthening the surrounding muscles of the lumbar-pelvic area help alleviate back pain.

Reduced stress. Stretching can help alleviate stress. It helps muscles to relax so they can absorb more nutrients and oxygen. Not only does this strengthen muscles, making them leaner and bigger, it also helps to decrease the buildup of toxins. Breathing, by itself, can also do wonders to help reduce stress.

When and How Much?

Just after your warmup on the stationary bike or treadmill, and just before your AH workout, you can stretch the muscles you'll be training that day, but for no longer than 2 to 5 minutes for each muscle group. When you stretch right before the workout, it stimulates bloodflow to the muscles.

You can also stretch *during* your workout, following a high-intensity set (one in which you work your muscles at 85 to 95 percent of their peak capacity). One stretch for 15 seconds will do. This will help maintain a constant delivery of oxygen and nutrients to the muscles.

Stretch for 2 to 5 minutes again after your AH workout, just as you did before you started. This will help your muscles relax and flush out any toxins that have accumulated. You'll also be less sore the next day, and your muscles will heal quicker.

What You Shouldn't Do

Never stretch a muscle or muscle group to the point where you feel pain. It's okay to feel a bit of a strain, but you shouldn't be clenching your jaw or feeling any discomfort in the joints surrounding the muscle.

Instead, slowly stretch the muscle to its full range of motion and add pressure by contracting the opposing muscle group. You can also add more pressure by leaning into the stretch with your body weight or engaging other muscles to increase the pressure on the muscle being stretched. For example, with the Triceps Stretch (see page 228), you can pull your elbow toward the center of your body while you squeeze the biceps to increase the pressure on the triceps.

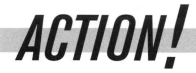

Action Hero: Adam Garcia

Career accomplishments: Adam has spent a lot of time moving his muscles. He's performed as a professional dancer in countless theater productions, both in his native country, Australia—he was in the opening ceremony of the Sydney Olympic Games—and in England, where he had roles in the stage versions of *Saturday Night Fever* and *Grease.* His big film breakthrough was as Kevin O'Donnell in *Coyote Ugly.*

Physical goals: Fat loss, muscle building, and improved stamina and endurance

Training program: What the Action Hero program is all about: weight lifting with a short cardiovascular activity right after the session

Results: Got him ready for the movie *Coyote Ugly*

Adam and I shared an interest in the same kind of music. So every session, Adam would bring in a "house music" CD to spice things up in the gym.

Adam was no stranger to working out, but he was like a sports car that had been sitting in the garage for too long. He was long overdue for a tune-up.

Once we got rolling, Adam took on the basic principles of the Action Hero

Action Hero Stretching Routine

Hold each of the stretches in the following routine for about 10 to 15 seconds. Remember, though, that when a stretched muscle wants to protect itself from being overstretched, or even ripped, it begins to contract. This is exactly the opposite of what you're trying to accomplish with stretching. To avoid this, apply a minimal amount of pressure and then increase it a little more every couple of seconds.

It's always a good thing to stretch, but it's also okay to forgo it every once in a while before, during, or after your AH workout. Just don't eliminate it completely. Personally, I do each of the following stretches once or twice, in sequence, two or three times per week.

training system. Time was an issue here, and I made it clear to him that diet was equally, if not more, important than working out. Especially if he intended to play a somewhat risqué scene as well as a dance-on-the-bar-without-a-shirt scene. We had to make sure he had the muscles to show off.

Our workouts consisted of very old-school sessions of hard-and-heavy lifting with sets of 6 to 8 reps in the 85 to 95 percent range of his capacity. The breakdown went like this: Day One—heavy back and biceps; Day Two—heavy chest and triceps; Day Three—heavy legs; Day Four—heavy shoulders and light arms. Right after each session he'd do an intense cardio session, or on a different day, he'd do a low to moderately intense aerobic session of up to 45 minutes. All in all, he was working out six times a week.

After he finished the movie, Adam went back to Australia. But when he came back for a short stay in Los Angeles, we met up to have one of the biggest and baddest burgers in L.A.

Hard and heavy lifting helps increase muscle tone. To decrease fat, restricting calorie intake helps. Even a mild, but frequent aerobic session helps stimulate the body to burn more calories (fat).

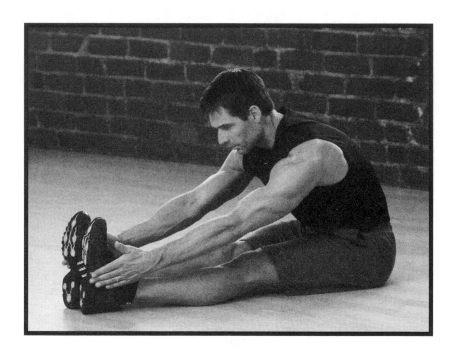

DOUBLE HAMSTRINGS

Sit on the floor with your legs together and place your hands on your thighs. Move them slowly toward your toes. If you can't reach your toes, it's not the end of the world, so don't hurt yourself trying. While doing this, keep your lower and upper back straight and don't hunch over.

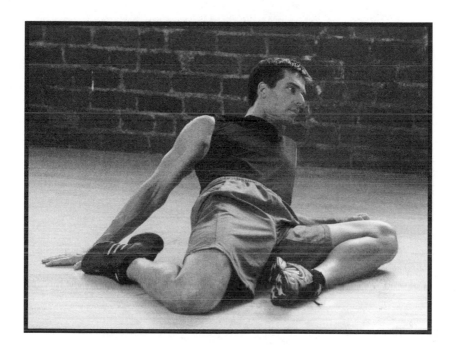

ONE-LEGGED QUAD/HIP FLEXORS

Lie on your side, leaning on your forearm, and bend the knee that's on the floor to a 90-degree angle. Pull this knee up until the thigh is perpendicular to your upper body. Situate the other leg, the one that's doing the stretching, in the same way, but pull it back. You can increase the intensity of the stretch by pulling one leg up more and the other back more. *Tip:* Squeeze the butt muscle of the leg being stretched.

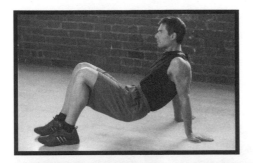

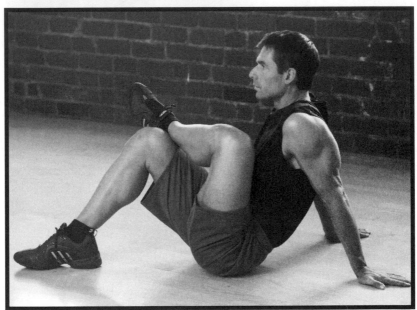

BUTT STRETCH

This is a tricky one to get into. Sit on the floor, leaning on your hands, feet on the floor with your knees bent. Lift your body up until you're balancing on your hands and feet with your butt off the floor. Lift one foot off the floor, cross that leg over the other, and place the foot on the other leg's thigh. Once you're in position, slowly lower yourself until your butt makes a touchdown on the floor. If the stretch is too intense, get out of it by reversing the procedure, and then place your foot a little farther away from your body. If the stretch doesn't feel like much, put your foot closer to your body.

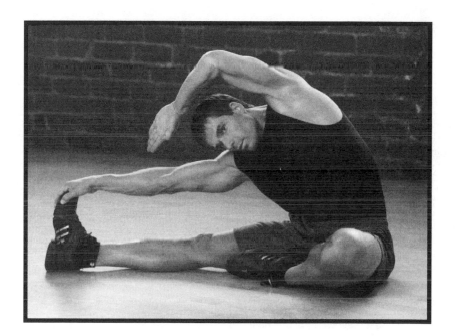

HAMSTRINGS/LATS AND QUADRATIS LUMBORUM STRETCH

Sit on the floor as you did for the Double Hamstrings stretch, legs together and straight out in front of you. Now pull in one leg and place the foot of the pulled-in leg against the inside thigh of the other leg. Hold on to the straight leg with the hand on that side. Slide your upper body sideways over the straight leg, and move the other arm over the side of your head. Feel the stretch.

WHAT TO DO WHEN YOU'RE SICK

You're feeling great, your workouts have been unbelievable, but now you're feeling a cold coming on. What to do?

In most cases, people feel they're still good to go for a regular workout, even if they have the sniffles.

Wrong!

If you're in the process of catching a cold, you *must* reduce the intensity of your workouts. It'll actually help your body to fight whatever demons are trying to take over.

When the body is in the beginning stages of a cold or flu, it uses its immune system to battle the bacteria or virus. Your body needs energy and micronutrients—such as vitamins, antioxidants, and minerals—to continue its battle.

If you work out while you're sick, you might feel fine but then an hour or two later, or maybe even the next morning, feel horrible. Here's why: Exercise requires energy, especially during the off days when muscles need to rebuild themselves. But our bodies need all that energy to stave off the effects of a cold or flu.

If we're sick and exercising at full capacity, our bodies end up being challenged on too many fronts.

Think of your immune system as a strong army. It has the situation under control as long as it's well-fed and armored. All of a sudden, though, the troops (the immune system) have to deliver nutrients and rebuilding material to the muscles after a workout, leaving themselves drastically undersupplied.

In many cases, this could have been avoided by actually helping the army get stronger by supplying it with proper ammunition (food, water, blood and oxygen, and rest).

So if you're sick with no significant fever, exercise at 50 percent of your maximum, and double the amount of rest between sets. Also, drink plenty of water, up your supplements, and go to bed a couple of hours earlier than usual. Trust me: You'll feel better the next day. During the past 9 months, I've gone up against "the enemy" at least a half-dozen times, and I have yet to catch a cold. So scale back on your workouts and let your body heal itself before you resume your normal intensity.

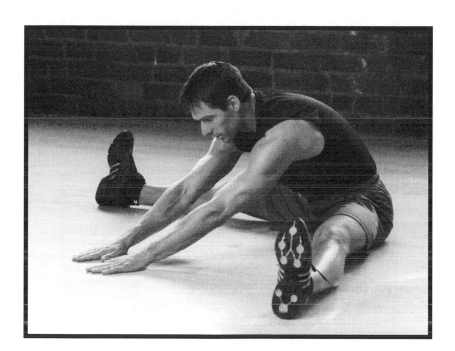

INNER THIGHS/HAMSTRINGS/
LAT STRETCH

Again, sit on the floor as you did for the hamstrings stretches. Gently open your legs sideways as far as your muscles allow. Put your hands on the floor in front of you and slowly reach forward. In an advanced stage of this stretch, you can spread your legs to almost a 180-degree angle and place your torso flat on the floor between them. For now, just try to reach a 90-degree angle with the legs, and put your elbows on the floor.

Here are some additional, muscle-specific stretches that you can add to the previous AH stretching routine, at your leisure.

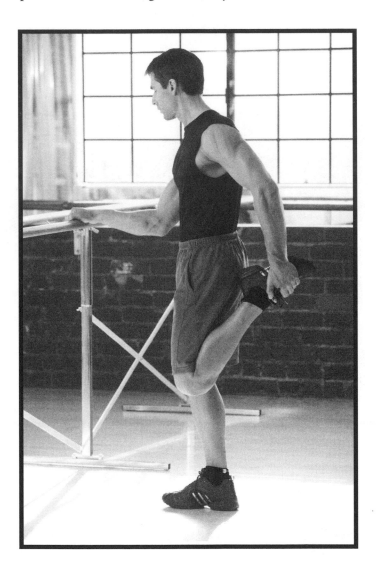

QUADS STRETCH

Stand on one leg, balancing yourself with one hand, while you reach behind you with the opposite hand, and hold on to the opposite foot. You can easily intensify the stretch by squeezing the butt muscle on the side of the quad that's being stretched. Do both quads.

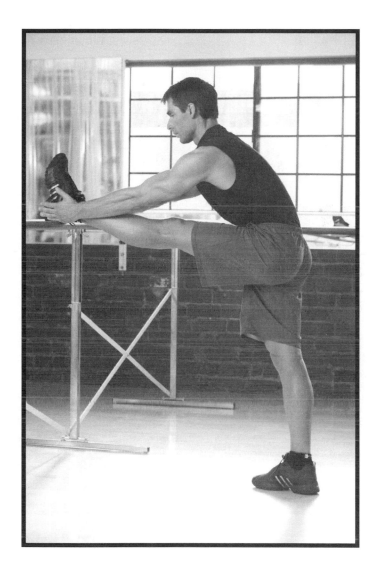

HAMSTRINGS STRETCH

Stand straight and place one leg on a bench or bar from a Smith machine. Rest both hands on the thigh that's being stretched and reach forward. Your flexibility will determine how far you can reach or how high the bench or bar should be.

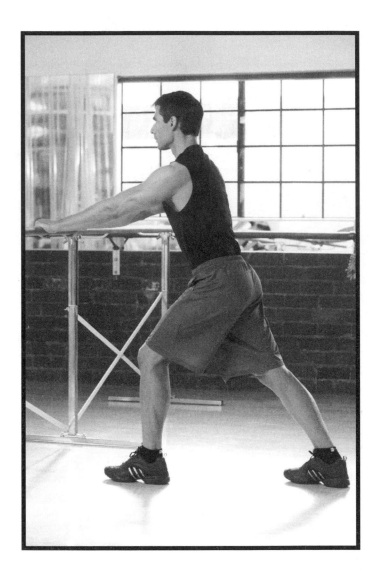

CALF STRETCH

Lean your hands against a machine or a wall, keeping your arms straight. Bend the knee of the front leg and keep the rear leg straight. Feet should be placed 1 to 2 feet apart, depending on your height. This will cause a mild stretch in the calves as a whole, including the gastrocnemius, soleus, and Achilles tendon. To intensify the stretch, place the rear foot a little farther away from the front foot. Switch sides and repeat with the other leg forward.

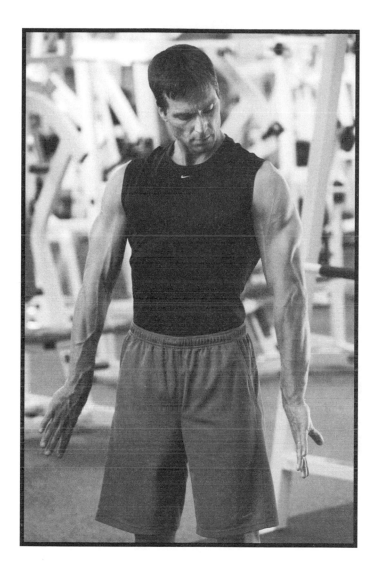

BICEPS STRETCH

Straighten both arms alongside your body and turn the palms of your hands outward. To increase the intensity of the stretch, contract your triceps and fully extend your elbows.

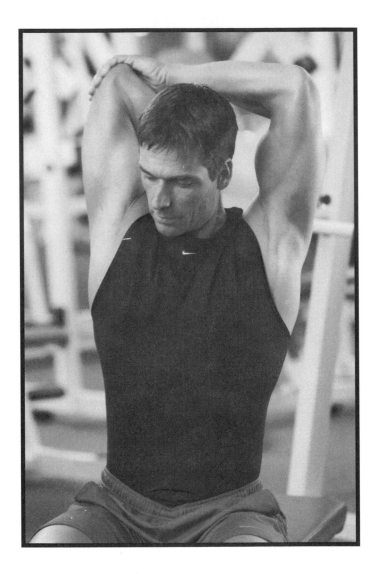

TRICEPS STRETCH

Lift one arm with the elbow bent until your hand reaches over your shoulder and touches your back. Squeeze your biceps and use the other hand to gently pull the elbow backward or toward the center of your body.

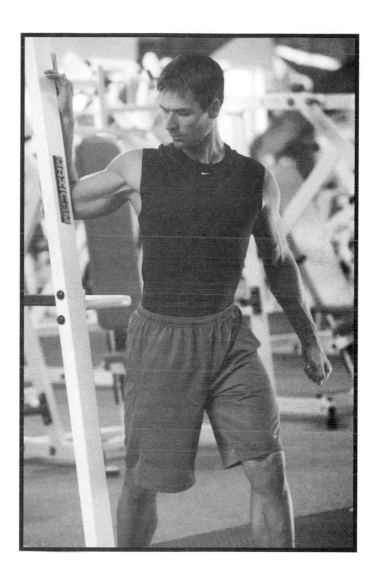

CHEST STRETCH

Find a doorpost or a machine that you can place your forearm against, as shown. Gently move your body forward to stretch the chest muscles. Switch sides and repeat.

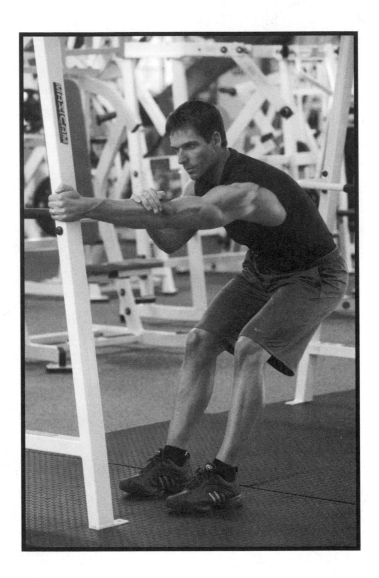

LAT STRETCH

Hold the vertical bar of a machine with your hand at stomach height and place your feet 12 inches or so from the machine. Lean back, extending your arm and upper body. Place the other hand on top of the straight arm. Move your upper body clockwise and counterclockwise to stretch the muscle at different angles and intensity levels.

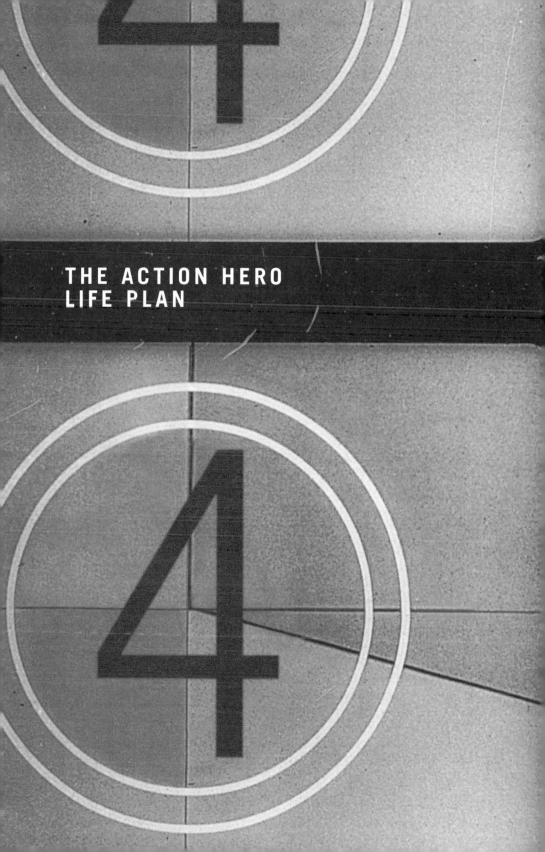

THE ACTION HERO
LIFE PLAN

9

MOTIVATION
MEDICINE

MOTIVATION IS THE POSITIVE, mental strength we call on to get a job done. Getting up every day, taking a shower, getting dressed, eating breakfast, and commuting to work all require motivation. We do these things without realizing that they require the same sort of effort and discipline as exercising and eating right. The only difference is that the daily habits have become a routine, and so we usually do them without too much effort.

And we do these things because we know the outcome. Work equals money. A healthy lifestyle with proper exercise and diet equals an Action Hero body.

Quite often motivation will surface when someone becomes inspired. You'd be motivated to quit smoking, for instance, if your doctor told you that if you don't stop now, today, you might be dead in a few years. That motivation to keep living and stop smoking is great, but I hope to catch you a little earlier in your life cycle.

Whatever your physical condition or habits, you'll call on that same inspiration to turn your body into an Action Hero's physique. And the reasons for doing so aren't too much different than the ones for, say, quitting smoking: reducing the risk of heart disease, lowering

CLIFF SHIEPE'S 3-WEEK TURNAROUND

"When I turned 34, I finally committed myself to getting in shape once and for all. Jørgen had told me about the 3-week turnaround and how the ultimate objective was to raise my basal metabolic rate. In fact, he had me circle the date (July 8) when this stage of the program would be complete. He told me up front not to expect too much until then, and that increasing my metabolic rate was more important than losing weight or gaining muscle.

"I won't lie here: Those first 3 weeks were hell. But during them I learned that Jørgen's program is best viewed as a process with distinct stages, the first being the 3-week turnaround. After that, I thought less about arriving somewhere and more about working in conjunction with my body. My role was clear: I had to commit to the process and understand that if I did my part as Jørgen instructed, my metabolic rate would increase, and that would carry me through the rest of the program. So I focused on breathing and mental preparation.

"Jørgen also had made it clear to me that the program is 70 percent food intake. I'd have to follow his dietary guidelines explicitly. He said I couldn't eat out and would have to start making my own food.

"Despite the 'hell' of those first 3 weeks, I never once was hungry or craved any particular food. I was able to commit to the plan because it was clear and simple. I loved being able to have some carbohydrates—two slices of bread with breakfast—after spending years on a high-protein diet. I was getting too much protein on that diet, I've since discovered.

cholesterol levels, and controlling chronic conditions such as diabetes and high blood pressure. But also, these reasons include more positive effects like maintaining an ideal weight, boosting energy levels, increasing strength, managing stress, and gaining a peppier outlook on life. Pick the ones that describe your situation and keep them in mind.

Once you've been inspired to follow this lifestyle, your Action Hero diet and exercise plan must also become routine if you want to succeed with them. Getting to that point is difficult, because our bodies and minds naturally resist anything new, particularly if it involves sweat, effort, and breaking old habits. But it is possible. Here are some tips to get you started.

"I quickly learned that the secret to success was preparation—plan ahead and execute. I can't stress enough how much mental energy you save when you understand what you must do to get where you want to go.

"I also began to focus on supporting my body with the appropriate amounts of supplements, water, and rest. I was totally surprised to learn firsthand how much of a difference vitamins and other supplements could make in one's life. Although in the past I always considered myself a disciplined person, after strenuous periods of diet and exercise, I'd hit a wall.

"Jørgen's first observation about me was right on the money. 'Cliff,' he said, 'the reason you're not getting the results you want is because you're doing too much.'

"Too much!

"By lowering the intensity of my cardio sessions to an inclined walk, for example, I can do much more without burning out. Jørgen changed my cardio program again during the third week. I went from two sessions a day for 30 minutes to two sessions a day for 45 minutes, and only one session on days I lifted weights.

"I really felt things kick in metabolically during week five. At that time I had also lost 15 pounds.

"Quite simply, this program has changed the quality of my life. I'm gaining back muscle while losing fat, and my metabolic rate is increasing even though I'm doing less intense cardio activity. I'm actually heading toward my Action Hero weight goal. I'd recommend Jørgen's plan to anyone."

In the beginning, you must put a lot of time and energy into your AH plan. The daily exercise will seem time-consuming, the diet will feel like a struggle, but never impossible. During the 3-week turnaround, you'll think that your life has become one endless trek to the gym, followed by a stint in the kitchen to cook up a decent meal. After the first enthusiasm wears off, you'll begin to wonder if the AH plan is really worth it.

The short answer, of course, is yes—it is. But also keep in mind that this resistance is normal and in fact a sign that your body and mind have taken notice of the new routine and are beginning to accept it.

Besides sticking faithfully to the program, one thing you can do while you work through this period is to stop thinking about what you don't want and start focusing on what you do. For example, rather than thinking, "I'm so tired I'm never going to make it through my workout today, much less want to cook dinner," think, "I'm tired, but I'll pull through and I'm on my way to building a healthy and great-looking body. I'll look forward to eating dinner after this." Whenever possible, replace those old, negative thoughts with positive ones.

Shoot down those excuses your mind will bring up, and believe me, they'll persist as you develop your new habits. Do you tell yourself you're too busy to exercise? The answer is to incorporate your routine into your daily schedule. Get up earlier, stop at the gym before you go home, or exercise during your lunch break. However you fit it in, make your workout as much a daily habit as brushing your teeth.

Is fatigue your excuse? It's likely that part of your problem is lack of exercise. Stop rushing around, getting through each day in crisis mode, and take the time to care for your body and your mind. Don't forget, your mind is a part of your body. You will benefit mentally, as well, from working out in the gym. It will reward you with more energy than you think possible. Tell yourself that you deserve to feel good, and that your AH routine will help you succeed with your other goals in life.

To stay motivated, you must give your body and mind a chance to adapt to the new routines, so go slowly at first. This is important, especially as a beginner. Work yourself through the stages program. Before you know it, you'll be on a roll and in high gear. If you push yourself too hard in the beginning, you'll get discouraged and quit before you've had a chance to reap the benefits.

Along the same lines, it's good to set goals to stay motivated. Keep them realistic, and set short-term goals on the way to your overall fitness goal. A good idea is to set daily and weekly goals. As a weekly goal, you might aim for working out 2 or 3 days out of the 7, and taking a walk every day after work on your off days. Whatever you decide, follow through with it. At the end of the week, review your goals and see how well you did. These weekly goals will help establish your AH routine as a daily habit. For a long-term goal, consider training for a fitness event or minitriathlon.

Getting bored is one of the fastest ways to lose motivation. Combat it by changing your routines. Work out according to the different cycles explained earlier in this book. Not only will this keep you interested, it will benefit your body by working different muscle groups at varying levels of intensity.

10 TIPS FOR STAYING FOCUSED

1. Take action every day by exercising and eating right.
2. Stick to the plan for at least 3 months. If, however, you fall off the wagon during this period, don't worry. You haven't failed. Just climb right back on again and continue your mission of becoming the AH that you want to be.
3. Accept resistance to change as part of the process.
4. Don't dwell on the perceived negatives. Focus on the positive aspects of the plan.
5. Slow down and make time to care for your body.
6. Set short-term goals on your way to long-term ones.
7. Vary your exercise routine and diet to avoid boredom.
8. Visualize yourself as fit and strong.
9. If you want, find others to exercise with, but always be accountable to yourself.
10. Reward your efforts when you reach a goal.

To keep your mind from sabotaging your efforts, put it to work visualizing how you want your body to look—bigger biceps, rock-hard abs, or whatever. Be realistic, though. You're not going to add 3 inches to your height or change a stocky build into a slim one. Concentrate on becoming the best "you" possible. Never forget—there's never best, but always better. You can always do better.

It helps, too, to involve your family or friends. The more people who know you're serious about your AH plan, the less opportunity you'll have to slack off. Be accountable to someone other than yourself. For example, you might want to join a basketball group at the gym a couple days a week as part of your aerobic activity. Once you're on the program,

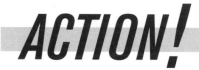

Action Hero: George Dzundza

Career accomplishments: George is a veteran character actor with a lot of work under his belt. Besides his role in *Crimson Tide,* he's appeared in *Dangerous Minds, Basic Instinct, No Way Out*, and *The Deer Hunter.* He's also appeared on stage and television, including the NBC sitcom *Jesse.*

Physical goals: Drastic weight loss in a short time and improved health, stamina, and strength

Training program: Aerobic activity integrated with a circuit weight-lifting program in conjunction with a virtually zero-calorie diet

Results: Mission accomplished! Weight loss of 60 pounds in just 6 weeks.

With George, I was faced with an extreme task for the first time: helping someone lose an insane amount of weight while simultaneously improving his health. In contrast with other Action Hero plans, this one didn't emphasize weight lifting, but rather moving around—as in lots and lots of aerobic activity.

In the beginning, George would do 20 minutes of aerobic activity in the early morning before breakfast. Later that day we met up in his gym for a weight-lifting session, which involved mostly the bigger muscle groups, such as legs, back, and chest. Then in the late afternoon, just before dinner, he'd do another aerobic session.

your family and friends will notice a difference in how you play and work. This should give you all the motivation you need.

Remember to reward yourself for your hard work, especially when you reach a long-term goal like dropping 10 pounds or staying on your diet for a full week, or following the instructions outlined in this book. Make the reward proportionate to the goal. This should be your newly acquired lifestyle, forever.

If you picked up this book purely out of desperation, know that if you read on and really stick to the program, you *will* lose weight and become stronger, more athletic, and healthier. Give it 3 good months, really working the program, before you even start thinking about going

Before long "Georgy" could do an hour of aerobics—usually walking on the treadmill while maintaining a heart rate of 130 to 135—in the morning and at night, in conjunction with an hour to an hour and a half of weight lifting a day.

As far as his diet was concerned, he had one meal replacement shake for breakfast, another for lunch, and some kind of lean fish with vegetables at night. He also took vitamins, minerals, and amino acids three to five times a day to ensure a steady supply of essential micronutrients. Obviously, he wasn't consuming enough food to supply him with that, so we had to give nature a helping hand.

During the first 10 days alone, Georgy lost 20 pounds. His weight loss was consistent, but not as dramatic, as the weeks passed. This was a good example of the weight-loss pattern I described elsewhere in this book.

We met the deadline, and Georgy was hired for the feature film *Crimson Tide*.

During his shoot we kept working out, and Georgy kept losing the weight and improving his health. The 14-hour workdays didn't seem to phase him. He became the inspiration of many young actors and members of the work crew on the set.

A severely restricted calorie intake works for maximum fat-burning and water loss. Be sure to compensate with an extensive amount of rest between workouts. Circuit training helps increase muscle tone and overall health.

in a different direction. Once you start the AH training system and the results begin to show, you'll be so motivated you won't want to fall back into your old bad habits. You'll be inspired to get in even better physical condition. You will become the best you can be.

Because I created this AH training system, I'm also its most devoted disciple. I practice what I preach. During the last 2 years, in particular, I've perfected the diet and training programs that are applicable to *any* healthy person—healthy enough to get to the gym and back home. If you follow the program faithfully, the results are guaranteed. Whether it's a well-proportioned body you want, overall good health, or a great sex life, they're all within reach as long as you stay the course. Even people with mild medical problems can turn their lives around and get healthy and strong once and for all.

Because I stick to the plan, I see a lot of positive short- and long-term results for myself. These keep me motivated, and they can work for you, too. Among other benefits, my productivity in life has increased 100 percent, I have more energy now than I've ever had, my immune system is stronger, and I've got six-pack abs and an overall low body fat percentage of 7 percent.

If any of this inspires you, then use it to begin the AH plan for yourself. Commit yourself to sticking with the plan, week by week, for 3 months. By doing so, you'll be working toward your goal in the fastest, most responsible way possible.

Believe and follow. It's that simple—and that difficult.

BIBLIOGRAPHY

Hatfield, Frederick C., *Hardcore Bodybuilding: A Scientific Approach*. Chicago: Contemporary Books, 1993.

Katch, Frank I., and William D. McArdle, *Introduction to Nutrition, Exercise, and Health*. Philadelphia/London: Lea and Febiger, 1993.

Sudy, Mitchell (supervising editor), *Personal Trainer Manual: The Resource for Fitness Instructors*. San Diego: American Council on Exercise, 1992.

Wharton, Jim and Phil, *The Whartons' Stretch Book*. New York: Times Books (Random House), 1996.

INDEX

Underscored page references indicate boxed text.
Boldface references indicate photographs.

A

Abdominals
about, 163
advanced exercises for
army-style situp, 169, **169**
bench crunch, 171, **171**
hanging leg raise, 168, **168**
knee lift, 170, **170**
exercises for beginners
crunch, 164, **164**
knee lift, 166, **166**
Rocky's, 167, **167**, **172**
side-to-side, 165, **165**
safety training tips, 172–73
Abs. *See* Abdominals
Action Heroes profiled
Adam Garcia, 216–17
Angelina Jolie, 64
Ben Affleck, 11–19, 19, 77–80
Billy Crudup, 92–93
Bridget Moynahan, 31
Cliff Shiepe, 71, 234–35
George Dzundza, 238–39
Jerry Bruckheimer, 9
Jerry O'Connell, 56
Josh Hartnett, 25
Robert Towne, 210
Action Hero program
diet plan for (*see* Diet)
as doable for everyone, 20–21, 240
emotional detachment and, 26
lifestyle change goals, 29–30

most challenging times, 43
motivation for, 233–40
overview of, 20–21, 24–27
quality of life with, 48–49
setting goals for, 29–30
stages of, 28–29
3-month commitment to, 237,
239, 240
tips for staying focused, 237
Activity, physical
caloric expenditure and, 27
overweight and, 46
Aerobic activity. *See also* Cardio test;
Cardiovascular exercises
Cart exercise, 22–23
for fat burning, 16, 19, 23
jogging as, 16
Affleck, Ben
career of, 18
diet designed for, 77–80
profile of, as Action Hero, 19
training program for, 11–19, 19
Age, quality of life and, 48–49
Air-conditioning, in gyms, 13, 177
Alcohol
avoiding, 40, 51
minimizing, 39
supplements and, 89
vitamin C and, 94
Allergies, food, supplements and, 89
American lifestyle and quality of life,
48

ABOUT THE AUTHOR

Jørgen de Mey has been called many things during his career as a personal trainer, including "a funny, happy drill sergeant," but one thing he's never been called is a slacker. Interested in total-body fitness even as a child in his native Holland, he began encouraging others to follow the fitness program he developed and that eventually evolved into the Action Hero training system. On the strength of the program, he competed successfully in bodybuilding events and coached his brother, Berry de Mey, to first place in the Mr. Europe bodybuilding competition and first place in the World Games in London. He established himself as a popular bodybuilder in the pro ranks. In 1988, he took third place in the Mr. Olympia competition, the most prestigious bodybuilding competition in the world.

Jørgen moved to Los Angeles when he was 23, where with the help of producer Jerry Bruckheimer he soon became a favorite of actors in need of a serious tune-up before films. He's trained Ben Affleck, Angelina Jolie, Jerry O'Connell, and Billy Crudup, among many others, and all with equal success.

Known for his straightforward, holistic approach to fitness, Jørgen combines practical, effective workouts with a sound nutrition plan and supplement regimen. He's followed the system himself for more than 20 years and has used it successfully to help not only movie stars, but people of all ages and physical conditions. He credits his success as a personal trainer to his unwavering self-discipline as well as a positive, moral, and ethical outlook on life.

"Even today I'm driven by other people's enthusiasm, and I'll always help them as much as I can to reach their goal," he says.

Now 38, Jørgen lives in Los Angeles with his wife, Angel, and two children, Vincent and Emma.

About the Cowriter

For more than 20 years, **Scott Hays**, M.A., has been a successful freelance writer. He has written for *TV Guide*, *Men's Health*, *Los Angeles Magazine*, *The Los Angeles Times*, *The Christian Science Monitor*, *Ad Age*, *The Miami Herald*, *Video Software Magazine*, and *The New York Daily News*. He also has authored or coauthored numerous nonfiction books for major publishers, including Warner Books and Barron's. His last book, *Built for Sex*, was published in 2005 by Rodale. Hays also teaches English and writing courses at several southern California colleges.